# Psychoanalytic Studies of Change

*Psychoanalytic Studies of Change* presents recent studies of the process and outcome of psychoanalytic therapy with an integrative perspective.

A recurrent challenge in the discussion of therapeutic outcome is the gap between empirical, quantitative studies, reporting results on a group level, and the clinician's interest in complex mechanisms of change presupposing microanalysis of dynamic interaction processes. This book bridges that gap via dynamic contributions from a variety of authors. Quantitative and qualitative studies are connected, epistemological and conceptual research is emphasized as specific domains, and in-depth clinical case studies are highlighted. The book comprises several new contributions to epistemology and conceptual research, as well as chapters discussing the challenge of combining qualitative and quantitative methods in studying process and outcome.

*Psychoanalytic Studies of Change* will not only meet a need specifically within psychoanalysis for up-to-date research but also provide an overview of the latest empirical research on psychoanalysis for a broader clinical and academic group of readers. It will appeal to psychoanalysts in practice and in training.

**Siri Erika Gullestad** is professor emeritus of clinical psychology at the University of Oslo, Norway. She is a training and supervising psychoanalyst and was awarded the Sigourney Award in 2019. An experienced teacher and supervisor, she is the author of numerous books and articles, including *The Theory and Practice of Psychoanalytic Therapy: Listening for the Subtext* (with Bjørn Killingmo, Routledge).

**Erik Stänicke** is professor of clinical psychology at the University of Oslo, Norway, and a training psychoanalyst. He is an experienced supervisor and teacher and is the author of numerous books and articles.

**Marianne Leuzinger-Bohleber** is professor emeritus of psychoanalysis at the University of Kassel, Germany. She is former director of the Sigmund-Freud-Institut in Frankfurt am Main, senior scientist at the University of Medicine in Mainz, a training and supervising analyst and author of numerous books and articles. She is the recipient of awards including the 2016 Sigourney Award and the IPA's Outstanding Scientific Achievement Award.

The International Psychoanalytical Association
Psychoanalytic Ideas and Applications Series
Series Editor Silvia Flechner
*IPA Publications Committee*

Natacha Delgado, Nergis Güleç, Thomas Marcacci, Carlos Moguillansky, Rafael Mondrzak, Angela M. Vuotto, and Gabriela Legoretta (consultant)

For more information, please visit https://www.routledge.com/The-International-Psychoanalytical-Association-Psychoanalytic-Ideas-and/book-series/KARNIPAPIA

"This book invites you to immerse yourself in recent psychoanalytic contributions to the study of psychic change and unconscious processes. Written by authoritative voices in the field, the chapters cover an impressive range of expertise, from clinical to statistical and developmental studies, and from neuroscience to a metacognitive analysis of self-reflection. An invaluable guide, this book skillfully navigates the complex terrain of contemporary psychoanalytic research, bridging multiple methodologies and perspectives."

**Ricardo Bernardi**,
*Professor Emeritus,*
*School of Medicine, Uruguay*


"This book on psychoanalytic studies of change processes presents groundbreaking psychoanalytic and interdisciplinary research on complex interactional processes that may hinder or promote development. It gives insight into the specifics of psychoanalysis as a scientific discipline and demonstrates how early experiences form the personality and how psychoanalytic processes may promote new development given its focus on deep emotional processes. The book is highly recommended for clinicians but also for researchers who want to understand better how enduring changes may develop."

**Sverre Varvin**,
*Professor Emeritus,*
*Oslo Metropolitan University, Norway*

# Psychoanalytic Studies of Change

## An Integrative Perspective

**Edited by**
**Siri Erika Gullestad, Erik Stänicke and**
**Marianne Leuzinger-Bohleber**

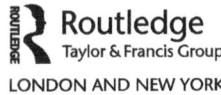

LONDON AND NEW YORK

Designed cover image: © Getty

First published 2024
by Routledge
4 Park Square, Milton Park, Abingdon, Oxon OX14 4RN

and by Routledge
605 Third Avenue, New York, NY 10158

*Routledge is an imprint of the Taylor & Francis Group, an informa business*

*British Library Cataloguing-in-Publication Data*
A catalogue record for this book is available from the British Library

ISBN: 9781032651927 (hbk)
ISBN: 9781032651903 (pbk)
ISBN: 9781032651934 (ebk)

DOI: 10.4324/9781032651934

Typeset in Palatino LT Std
by codeMantra

# Contents

# Series Editor's Foreword

The Publications Committee of the International Psychoanalytic Association is pleased to continue with the present volume in the series "Psychoanalytic Ideas and Applications." The objective of the series is to focus on the scientific output of significant authors whose works are outstanding contributions to the development of the psychoanalytic field. The series aims to set out relevant ideas generated during the history of psychoanalysis which deserve to be known and discussed by psychoanalysts in our time.

The relationship between psychoanalytic ideas and their applications needs to be put forward from the perspective of theory, clinical practice, and research, to maintain the validity for contemporary psychoanalysis. The Publications Committee's goal is to share these new ideas with the psychoanalytic community and with professionals in related disciplines, to expand their knowledge and generate a productive exchange between the text and the reader. As such, the IPA Publications Committee is pleased to publish the book *Psychoanalytic Studies of Change: An Integrative Perspective*, edited by Siri Erika Gullestad, Erik Stänicke, and Marianne Leuzinger-Bohleber.

As the editors highlight:

> A recurrent challenge in the discussion of therapeutic outcome is what has been called a "gap" between empirical, quantitative studies, reporting results on a group level, and the clinician's interest in complex mechanisms of change presupposing microanalysis of dynamic interaction processes. Attempting to bridge this gap, this book presents recent studies of process and outcome of psychoanalytic therapy with an integrative perspective. Quantitative and qualitative studies are connected, epistemological and conceptual research are emphasized as specific domains, and in-depth clinical case studies are highlighted.

This book integrates the following topics within which excellent chapters are included both from the clinical theoretical point of view and articles related to research. The book is organized into four parts: "Process and

Outcome," "Conceptual Studies," "Prevention," and "In Search of Methods." They cover a wide spectrum of authors and topics that will enlighten the reader due to their depth and innovative approaches. The authors of each chapter are outstanding psychoanalysts who have devoted much of their work to deepening the issues presented within this book. It will undoubtedly be of interest to the psychoanalytic community, as well as the wide range of psychoanalysts and neighboring fields of interest in theoretical, clinical, and research topics.

Silvia Flechner
*Series Editor*
*Chair, IPA Publications Committee*

# Preface

We are pleased to present this book which was initiated by the Research Committee of the International Psychoanalytic Association (IPA).

Historically, psychoanalysis had a difficult time promoting research, Robert N. Emde and Peter Fonagy stated in the late 1990s. Although psychoanalysis began by generating an extraordinarily innovative body of knowledge, it grew in isolation from universities and mainly focused on one method of enquiry, namely, the psychoanalytic situation (Emde & Fonagy, 1997, 643). Although since the 1920s analysts also attempted to study the outcomes of psychoanalysis empirically, they remained rather on the fringes of the psychoanalytic community (see, e.g., Leuzinger-Bohleber et al., 2020). During the 1990s something changed, marked by several important events: a research training program for promoting psychoanalytic research, led by Peter Fonagy, opened for fellows from all over the world. Also in the 1990s, *The International Journal of Psychoanalysis* under the leadership of David Tuckett initiated an in-depth discussion about scientific standards for publication of case studies. Moreover, plans were made for "open door reviews," enabling the dissemination of psychoanalytic research, led by Horst Kächele and Marianne Leuzinger-Bohleber. And – not least – the Joseph Sandler Psychoanalytic Research Conference was established with the specific aim of stimulating dialogue between clinicians and researchers. The Sandler conference has since been an annual event, first in London, then in Frankfurt, then as an event circulating between Latin America, United States, and Europe. In 2022, the Sandler conference – titled *In Search of Change: Psychoanalytic Process and Outcome* – took place in Oslo, Norway. The contributions of this volume are based on papers delivered at this conference. However, the book is in no way a conference proceeding. Conference papers have been significantly elaborated and the book also comprises several new contributions to epistemology and conceptual research, as well as chapters discussing the challenge of combining qualitative and quantitative methods in studying change.

The Sandler conference in Oslo was hosted by the Norwegian Psychoanalytic Society in collaboration with the Department of Psychology, University of Oslo. While psychoanalysis in many countries grew in isolation from universities, the University of Oslo has a vital psychoanalytic research tradition initiated by Harald Schjelderup, Norway's first psychology professor, who was also psychoanalyst – he got his professorship in 1928. Schjelderup introduced for the university the psychoanalytic *Tiefenpsychologie* – the "depth psychological method" – as a specific research method aimed at studying unconscious fantasy and conflict. The psychoanalytic method provides us access to an understanding of the human mind that is *specific*: "Data" from the therapy room – our clinical "laboratory" – give a different picture of how a traumatic event like childhood sexual abuse is handled by the human psyche, rather than, for example, data from memory research. Such data represent a supplement to other research methods and are necessary for a full understanding of personality as well as of psychic suffering. Schjelderup's "programme" consisted also in integrating psychoanalytic knowledge as part of general psychology – psychoanalysis indeed needs a dialogue with other scientific fields. It is question of a double-edged epistemological stance: on the one hand, psychoanalysis represents a specific depth psychological research method necessary for capturing unconscious aspects of the mind that are not accessible by other methods. On the other hand, psychoanalysis needs to be in dialogue with other scientific disciplines, like developmental psychology, memory research, cultural studies, philosophy, and neuroscience. It needs to correct its assumptions, for example developmental studies have demonstrated that some psychoanalytic assumptions are not tenable. The dialogue between different fields of enquiry is enriching for both parts. Most importantly, we think the dialogue between psychoanalysis and academia is essential for the future of psychoanalysis.

The theme of this book is "change." As an academic psychoanalyst, Schjelderup in the 1950s realized the need for empirical documentation of the effects of psychoanalytic treatment. His studies of the lasting, personality-changing processes of psychoanalytic treatment (Schjelderup, 1955, 1956) were pioneering in highlighting how psychoanalysis results in qualitative changes in, for example, the individual's experience of self and reality. Schjelderup's unique position and influence on Norwegian psychology and psychoanalysis was probably also due to his role as a leader of the resistance movement at the university during Germany's nazi-occupation of Norway during WW2. Both in the resistance fight and in his professional discussions with IPA, Schjelderup came forward as a person with exceptional integrity, courage, and intellectual strength (see also Nilsen, 2011; Anthi & Haugsgjerd, 2013; Nilsen, 2013).

The Department of Psychology, with its leader Bjørn Lau, agreed to host the Sandler Conference in Oslo in 2022. To maintain psychoanalytic and dynamic psychology as a clinical and theoretical discipline within this department has been a history of continual fight – sometimes hard disputes. As a leader, Lau acknowledges that psychoanalytic studies represent an important part of the broad science of psychology, stretching from experimental laboratory research and social psychology to hermeneutic interpretation of culture and studies from the clinical "laboratory." Our most heartfelt thanks go to Bjørn Lau.

Our warm thank you to the president of the IPA, Harriet Wolfe and her administration for their acknowledgment, respect, and support of research as a vital activity of IPA and to the Research Committee of IPA who, in different ways, have contributed to create the program presented at the conference. Our profound thanks also go to the administrative secretary of the Norwegian Psychoanalytic Society, Anne Kullebund. Without her outstanding professional capacity for arranging big events – Anne has for many years been part of teams organizing Olympic games in diverse countries – the Sandler 2022 conference had come to nothing.

Siri Erika Gullestad, Erik Stänicke and
Marianne Leuzinger-Bohleber
August 2023

## References

Anthi, P. & Haugsgjerd, S. (2013). A note on the history of the Norwegian Psycho-analytic Society from 1933 to 1945. International Journal of Psychoanalysis, 94(4), 715–724.

Emde, R. N. & Fonagy, P. (1997) An Emerging Culture For Psychoanalytic Research?. International Journal of Psychoanalysis, 78, 643–651.

Leuzinger-Bohleber, M., Arnold, S. & Solms, M. (Hrsg.) (2020). Outcome research and the future of psychoanalysis. London: Routledge.

Nilsen, H.F. (2011). The history of psychoanalysis in Norway. In P. Loewenberg & N.L. Thompson (Red.), 100 years of the IPA. The centenary history of International Psychoanalytical Association, 1910–2010 (pp. 140–148). London: Karnac Books.

Nilsen, H.F. (2013). Resistance in therapy and war. Psychoanalysis before and during the Nazi occupation of Norway 1933–1945. International Journal of Psychoanalysis, 94, 725–746.

Schjelderup, H. (1955). Lasting effects of psychoanalytic treatment. Psychiatry, 18, 109–133.

Schjelderup, H. (1956). Personality-changing processes of psychoanalytic treatment. Acta Psychologica, 12, 47–64.

# Contributors

**Carolina Altimir** is assistant professor and Director of Graduate Studies and Research Faculty of Psychology, Universidad Alberto Hurtado. She is a clinical psychologist and psychotherapist, practicing in private practice.

**Gilles Ambresin** is senior lecturer and Privat-Docent at the Faculty of Biology and Medicine, Lausanne University Hospital. He is an associate member of the Swiss Psychoanalytic Society.

**Werner Bohleber** is a psychoanalyst in private practice in Frankfurt am Main. He is training and supervising analyst and former President of the German Psychoanalytical Association. In 2007, he received the Mary S. Sigourney Award.

**Nicole Cain** is associate professor in the Graduate School of Professional Psychology, Rutgers University, the State University of New Jersey.

**Eve Caligor** is clinical professor of Psychiatry, Columbia University Vagelos College of Physicians and Surgeons.

**John F. Clarkin** is clinical professor of Psychology in Psychiatry, Weill Medical College of Cornell University. He serves as the Head of Faculty of the Research Training Program of the International Psychoanalytic Association.

**Stephan Doering** is professor of psychoanalysis and psychotherapy at the Medical University of Vienna. He is a psychoanalyst at the Vienna Psychoanalytic Society.

**Constanza Duhalde** is professor at the University of Buenos Aires and associate professor of at the University of Belgrano. She is psychoanalyst at the Argentine Society of Psychoanalysis.

**Siri Erika Gullestad** is professor emeritus of clinical psychology at the University of Oslo. She is a training and supervising analyst and former president of the Norwegian Psychoanalytic Society. In 2019, she received the Mary S. Sigourney Award. She is currently Chair of IPA Research Committee.

**Alexandra M. Harrison** is associate professor in psychiatry at the Harvard Medical School, Cambridge Health Alliance, and Core Faculty of the Fellowship in Early Relational Health at University of Massachusetts Chan Medical School. She is a training and supervising analyst in child and adolescent and adult psychoanalysis at the Boston Psychoanalytic Society and Institute.

**Stephan Hau** is professor of clinical psychology at Stockholm University and a psychoanalyst at the Swedish and German Psychoanalytic Society. He is Editor-in-Chief of the Scandinavian Psychoanalytic Review. He is currently Co-chair of IPA Research Committee.

**Cecilie Hillestad Hoff** is a PhD candidate at the Department of Psychology at the University of Oslo. She is a psychoanalyst at the Norwegian Psychoanalytic Society.

**Vanina Huerin** is associate professor at the University of Buenos Aires.

**Juan Pablo Jiménez** is professor emeritus at the University of Chile. He is a psychoanalyst at the Chilean Psychoanalytic Association, where he has been a former president. He has also been a former president of the Latin American Psychoanalytic Federation.

**Rogerio Lerner** is associate professor at the Institute of Psychology with subsidiary link with the Department of Psychiatry of the Faculty of Medicine of the University of São Paulo. He is an associate member at the Brazilian Psychoanalytic Society of Sao Paulo. In 2019, he received the Psychoanalytic Research Exceptional Contribution Award. He is currently Co-chair of IPA Research Committee.

**Marianne Leuzinger-Bohleber** is professor emeritus for psychoanalysis at the University of Kassel, senior professor at the University of Medicine in Mainz, and former director of the Sigmund-Freud-Institut in Frankfurt. She is training analyst of the German psychoanalytical Association (DPV). She received the Mary S. Sigourney Award (2016), the Haskell Norman Prize for Excellence in Psychoanalysis (2017), the Robert S. Wallerstein Fellowship (2022–2027), and the IPA Outstanding Scientific Achievement Award (2023).

**Elizabeth J. Levey** is assistant professor of psychiatry at Harvard Medical School MD. She is a graduate of the adult psychoanalytic program and a member of the faculty at the Chicago Psychoanalytic Institute; she is also an advanced candidate in child psychoanalysis.

**Steinar Lorentzen** is professor emeritus in psychiatry at the University of Oslo, Norway. He is a psychoanalyst at the Norwegian Psychoanalytic Society.

**Yamil Quevedo** is assistant professor of psychiatry at the University of Chile and postdoctoral researcher at the Millennium Institute for Research on Depression and Personality (MIDAP).

**Clara Raznoszczyk Schejtman** is professor and director of research programs at the University of Buenos Aires and Head Professor of Child and Adolescent Clinical Psychology at the University of Belgrano. She is a training analyst and a member of the Argentine Psychoanalytic Association.

**Mark Solms** is professor of neuropsychology at the University of Cape Town. He is training and supervising analyst at the South African Psychoanalytical Society, where he was former president. In 2011, he received the Sigourney award and in 2017 the IPA's Outstanding Scientific Achievement Award. He is currently Director of APsaA's Science Department.

**Hanne Strømme** is associate professor of clinical psychology at the University of Oslo (UiO). She is psychoanalyst at the Norwegian Psychoanalytic Society.

**Erik Stänicke** is professor of clinical psychology at the University of Oslo, and training analyst at the Norwegian psychoanalytic society, where he has also been former president. He is currently Co-chair of IPA Research Committee.

**Line Indrevoll Stänicke** is associate professor of clinical psychology at the University of Oslo and senior researcher at the Lovisenberg Hospital in Oslo, Norway. She is a psychoanalyst at the Norwegian Psychoanalytic Society.

**Ines Vardy** is a PhD and child psychiatrist. She is psychoanalyst at the Argentina Psychoanalytic Association.

**María Pía Vernengo** is professor at the University of Buenos Aires and associate professor of at the University of Belgrano.

# Introduction

## In search of change

*Siri Erika Gullestad, Erik Stänicke*
*and Marianne Leuzinger-Bohleber*

> I'm actually embarrassed to say.... Actually, I am now quite satisfied with my-
> self, as I am now.... That I can love and have fun, think and understand.... And
> that I could fight my way out of the whole mud.... It's quite good that way,
> I can love and be loved and above all, just take a break …
>
> (Mr. P.)

This is how a patient of the MODE study expressed himself at the end of an analytic session in the 4th year of his psychoanalysis. In a contemplative way, he reflects on what for him are the most important results of his psychoanalysis. While on the one hand his formulations recall Freud's famous characterization of the goals of psychoanalysis, "the aim of the treatment will never be anything else but the practical recovery of the patient, the restoration of his ability to lead an active life and of his capacity for enjoyment" (Freud, 1904, p. 253), often translated as "capacity for love and work". On the other hand, the citation also describes very specific, individual issues: Mr. P. can again "think and comprehend," be proud of the fact that he has "fought his way out of the mud," and "can also just take a break like that." The now nearly 30-year-old student had sought therapeutic help four years ago in a desolate mental and psychosocial state after a serious suicide attempt. He had completely withdrawn into his own, nearly autistic world, cutting off his studies, and virtually all of his social relationships, spending his days mostly in bed in a dark room alone, after nights of extremely disturbed sleep, terrible nightmares, and acute suicidal impulses (Leuzinger-Bohleber, 2023).

Such formulations of analysands may sound familiar to many analytic readers. On the basis of their distinctive life and trauma story, analysands describe in their very own words, images, and metaphors which changes took place during their psychoanalytic treatment, which turning-points were decisive for them, and how these transformed the basic melody of their psyche, the idiosyncratic structures, and processes of their micro-worlds. Are analysts therefore right when they insist that processes of change in psychoanalysis cannot be scientifically researched, i.e., "objectified" in any way, checked for their intersubjective truth content, or even "measured" in

DOI: 10.4324/9781032651934-1

any way, but can only be told? Should psychoanalysis refuse any form of extra-clinical research and remain in the realm of subjectivity of the individual case?

In this brief introduction, we will present some reflections on the epistemological, historical, and societal background of psychoanalysis that frames all the different perspectives within the pluralism of psychoanalytic research today. It is within this framework that we briefly place the individual contributions of this volume, in order to provide the reader an initial overview.

### Psychoanalysis as a plural science: some historical remarks

What did Freud mean when he defined psychoanalysis as a specific "science of the unconscious"? (see, for example, Whitebook, 2017). As a young man, Freud was known to have been very interested in philosophy and the humanities before turning to the natural sciences with a strikingly intensive emotional reaction. He was then working in medical neurological research in the laboratory at Ernst Brücke's Physiological Institute, where he encountered a strictly positivist understanding of science that attracted him throughout his life. As we know, Freud nevertheless later turned away from the neurology of his time, recognizing the limits of the methodological possibilities for investigating psychic processes in this discipline. With the *Interpretation of Dreams*, the birth document of psychoanalysis, he defined it as "pure psychology." However, he continued to see himself as a physician who observed clinical phenomena like a natural scientist. In his recent Freud biography, Joel Whitebook (2017) emphasizes that Freud's desire for precise "empirical" testing of hypotheses and theories protected him from his own tendency toward wild speculation (Whitebook, 2010). This enabled him, as a "philosophical physician," to develop a new "'depth-psychology', a theory of the mental unconscious" (Freud, 1926, p. 248. For a discussion of the epistemology of psychoanalysis, see Stänicke et al., 2020).

The aim of psychoanalytic treatment, says Freud, is to strengthen the ego in relation to the superego, facilitating appropriation of unconscious driving forces – "where id was, there ego shall be" (Freud, 1933, p. 80) – thus allowing for a more lucid self-knowledge, a vision of enlightenment. As emphasized by the philosopher Jürgen Habermas (1969), psychoanalysis is guided by an interest in *emancipatory knowledge*. However, Freud's conception of rationality is an expanded one. As emphasized already by Heinz Hartmann (1939) in a discussion of the psychoanalytic conception of health, "the most rational attitude does not necessarily constitute an optimum for the purpose of adaptation (...) The rational must incorporate the irrational as an element in its design" (Hartmann, 1939, pp. 9–10). On this background, Whitebook (2017, p. 12) places Freud in the tradition of so-called dark enlightenment" – his theoretical task consisted in confronting the irrational in order to integrate it into a fuller and richer conception of reason. Science, according to Freud, is a mode of thought and practice that befits the finite human mind – it is an institutionalized practice based on the recognition of "the human animal's innate tendency omnipotently to deny reality – the human penchant for magical thinking – *and it constitutes the methodological struggle against it*" (Whitebook, 2017, p. 398).

Institutionally, Freud's self-understanding of psychoanalysis as a *specific* science was a key to the success story of psychoanalysis. As is well known, Freud was still considering in 1909 whether it would be beneficial for the future of the young discipline to join August Forel's medical organization "Medical Psychology and Psychotherapy" or even the Order for Ethics and Culture. Fortunately, however, on New Year's Eve 1910, he decided to found his own psychoanalytic organization, the International Psychoanalytic Association (see, amongst others, Falzeder, 2010, Leuzinger-Bohleber, 2021). This ensured institutionally – and methodologically – the independence of psychoanalysis as a scientific discipline, to which Freud always adhered thereafter. It was not at all desirable for psychoanalysis "to be swallowed up by medicine," but that it "as 'depth psychology,' a theory of the mental unconscious, it can become indispensable to all the sciences which are concerned with the evolution of human civilization and its major institutions such as art, religion, and the social order" (Freud, 1926, p. 248). In this context, his detailed case histories proved crucial. He himself noted that they were to be read more like great literature than like results of medical research.

In the 1960s, Habermas (1969) spoke about the "scientific self-misunderstanding" of psychoanalysis, referring to Freud's lifelong hope that the clinical insights of psychoanalysis could also be "objectively" verified with "hard" natural scientific methods. His distinction between psychoanalysis pursuing an "emancipatory interest in knowledge" and behavior therapy, which was committed to a "technical interest in knowledge" (Habermas, 1969), was echoed by an entire generation. As a critical-hermeneutic method, psychoanalysis gained wide influence – for highlighting unconscious sources of psychic and psychosomatic suffering, for elucidation of extreme ideologies (Reich, 1933; Fromm et al., 1936; Adorno et al., 1950; Bohleber, 2010; Gullestad, 2017), as well as for social-psychological and cultural-critical analyses (e.g., Mitscherlich, 1963). A rich interdisciplinary exchange with philosophy, sociology, literary sciences, the humanities, as well as with film and art ensured, in many places, the social acceptance of psychoanalysis in those times. At the same time, empirical and especially quantitative measurement research or dialogue with the natural sciences was judged by many to be naïve and inappropriate to psychoanalysis, even harmful. For example, the innovative attempt of the Ulm group in Germany around Herbert Thomä and Horst Kächele to tape record and systematically study psychoanalytic treatments, to enable dialogue with empirical psychotherapy research, was met by devaluation and open rejection by a large part of the psychoanalytic community (see also Leuzinger-Bohleber, 2021).

Now the times are changing! Increasingly, it is realized that if psychoanalysis wants to remain in the world of science, we must take account of the new demands for demonstrating *evidence*. Is psychoanalytic treatment cost efficient? Could shorter treatment formats be as efficient? In this context, we want to highlight some characteristics of the status of science in our present day society. Over the past 300 years, Western societies have devoted a large part of their resources to acquiring, expanding, and verifying their knowledge. In the last century, the industrial society has changed into a *knowledge society*. A first component of the changes in the sciences concerns *differentiation*. As Hermann von Helmholtz noted 100 years ago, each individual researcher is increasingly forced to address *narrower and narrower* questions using ever more *specific* methods. The days of the universal genius are bygone: Today's scientists are mostly highly specialized experts with a very limited knowledge of adjacent fields (von Helmholtz, 1896, cited in Weingart, 2002, p. 703). They depend on networking internationally, intergenerationally, and interdisciplinarily to investigate complex problems. In connection with this process of differentiation, the *criteria* of "science" and "scientific truth" in the respective scientific disciplines, both in the natural sciences and the humanities, have also changed and become more specific: The idea of a unified science (Einheitswissenschaft) based on the experimental design of classical physics (and the double-blind experiment that emerged from it) turned out to be a myth: We live in a time of "plurality of sciences" (Hampe, 2003).

A second feature of the changes in psychoanalysis' attitude toward research concerns the *relationship between science and society*. Today's scientific disciplines – and thus also psychoanalysis – are in constant, accelerated, global competition at various levels. For example, the pragmatic relevance of research is constantly evaluated by societal funders and political interest groups, which are gaining more and more influence, e.g., through the funding of research projects. In this sense, science is increasingly losing its autonomy. *Science is becoming politicized – politics is becoming scientific*. It is precisely in this context that the communication of methods and results of scientific studies is crucial, and with it the ability to put them into narratives that are comprehensible to lay people, despite all their specificities. Albert Einstein was a great storyteller: without this ability, it is questionable whether the theory of relativity would have had such a broad social impact. The same is still true for Sigmund Freud. "The most important characteristic of today's societies is the competition for trust" says the sociologist Peter Weingart: "When trust is earned, it is priceless and science should be urgent not to lose trust. Therefore, efforts to produce trust and credibility are ever increasing" (Weingart, 2002, p. 706; our translation). Moreover, which scientists are most likely to be trusted depends to a large extent on their *credibility as conveyed by the media*. Media therefore becomes a relevant social factor for which there is now competition in politics as well as in the public sphere. Thus, a challenge for psychoanalysis today is to present its research in narratives that can be trusted.

Our book presents several new narratives and original conceptual integrations. Mark Solms, based on neuroscience, tells us a fresh story about how to understand the change mechanism of the talking cure (Chapter 9); Werner Bohleber conveys an integrative comprehension of the role of self-agency and self-reflection in change (Chapter 8); Line Stänicke, based on innovative methodology for studying self-harm, which also provides new concepts, presents lively prototypes of young women harming themselves (Chapter 14); Siri Erika Gullestad argues convincingly for affirmation as part of therapeutic action (Chapter 10); and Erik Stänicke provides an in-depth reflection on the epistemological position of our discipline, arguing psychoanalysis can be situated in a long tradition within epistemology that goes back to the philosopher Immanuel Kant (Chapter 7). The demand for *evidence* of psychoanalytic treatment is addressed by several chapters. The ongoing international MODE study, speaking to the question of intensity of treatment sessions, is presented by Marianne Leuzinger-Bohleber and Gilles Ambresin (Chapters 2 and 3); John Clarkin and his colleagues analyze outcome and processes of change in Transference Focused Therapy, illustrated with clinical material (Chapter 1); and Steinar Lorentzen (Chapter 6) presents results of, for example, impressive RCT and naturalistic studies of short and long analytic group treatment. Outcome studies raise the question of valid diagnostics, engagingly highlighted by Stephan Doering (Chapter 5). Juan Pablo Jimenez and Yamil Quevedo offer a compelling overview of the relevance of epigenetics for therapeutic change (Chapter 5). Moreover, *differentiation* of methods is amply illustrated in our book. New methods for studying mother-infant interaction are inspiringly illustrated by Rogerio Lerner (Chapter 11), Clara Schejtman (Chapter 12), and Alexandra Harrison and Elizabeth Levey (Chapter 13) presents methods used in preventive programs enabling change in destructive interaction patterns. Recent innovative development in methodology allowing for microanalytic examination of therapeutic dialogues is presented by Juan Pablo Jimenez and his group (Chapter 17). Cecilie Hillestad Hoff (Chapter 15) discusses what psychoanalysis can learn from qualitative and quantitative psychotherapy research, yet steer clear of some of its pitfalls. Innovative methods for capturing processes of therapist learning are discussed by Hanne Strømme and Stephan Hau (Chapter 16).

Our book aims at balancing between today's demand for an evidence base for every treatment modality, in an often critical and competitive – sometimes even hostile – environment and, as emphasized by Mark Solms, the need to recognize the complexities that must be taken into account to obtain a valid picture of what "outcome" means when the subject of change is something as complex and intangible as the life of the mind.

## References

Adorno, T.W., Frenkel-Brunswick, E., Lewinson, D.J. & Sanford, R.N. (1950). *The authoritarian personality*. New York: Harper.

Bohleber, W. (2010). *Destructiveness, intersubjectivity and trauma: The identity crisis of modern psychoanalysis*. London: Karnac Books.

Falzeder, E. (2010). *Die Gründungsgeschichte der IPV und der Berliner Ortsgruppe*. Vortrag auf der Tagung der DPG und DPV: 100 Jahre Internationale Psychoanalytische Vereinigung (IPV) – 100 Jahre institutionalisierte Psychoanalyse in Deutschland, Berlin, 6.3.2010.

Freud, S. (1904) Freud's psycho-analytic procedure. *SE* 7.

Freud, S. (1926). The question of lay analysis. *SE* 20.

Freud, S. (1933). New introductory lectures on psychoanalysis. *SE* 22.

Fromm, E., Horkheimer, M., Mayer, H. & Marcuse, H. (1936). *Autorität und Familie*. Paris: Felix Alcan.

Gullestad, S.E. (2017). Anders Behring Breivik, master of life and death: Psychodynamics and political ideology in an act of terrorism. *International Forum of Psychoanalysis 26*(4), 1–10.

Habermas, J. (1969). *Erkenntnis und Interesse*. Frankfurt: Suhrkamp.

Hampe, M. (2003). Pluralism of sciences and the unity of reason. In M. Leuzinger-Bohleber, A.U. Dreher & J. Canestri (Hrsg.), *Pluralism or unity? Methods of research in psychoanalysis* (S. 45–63). London: International Psychoanalytical Association.

Hartmann, H. (1939). Psychoanalysis and the concept of health. In *Essays on ego psychology*. New York: International Universities Press, 1964, pp. 3–18.

Leuzinger-Bohleber, M. (2021). Psychoanalyse als plurale Wissenschaft des Unbewussten. *Allgemeine Zeitschrift für Philosophie, 46*(2), 253–267.

Leuzinger-Bohleber, M. (2023): Depression – eine Krankheit des Ideals und des Traumas. In: *Psychoanalyse in Europa*. Bulletin, Nr. 76: 208–223 (article printed in German, English and French).

Mitscherlich, A. (1963). *Auf dem Veg zur Vaterlosen Gesellschaft. Ideen zur Sozialpsychologie*. München: R.Piper & Co Verlag.

Reich, W. (1933). *Massenpsychologie des Fascismus*. Copenhagen: Verlag für Sexualpolitik.

Stänicke, E., Zachrisson, A. & Vetlesen, A.J. (2020). The Epistemological Stance of Psychoanalysis: Revisiting the Kantian Legacy. *The Psychoanalytic Quarterly, 89*(2): 281–304.

Weingart, P. (2002). The moment of truth for science. The consequences of the 'knowledge society' for society and science. *EMBO Reports, 3*, 703–706.

Whitebook, J. (2010). *Sigmund Freud – A philosophical physician*. Vortrag bei der 11. Joseph Sandler Research Conference: Persisting shadows of early and later trauma. Frankfurt a.M., 7.2.2010.

Whitebook, J. (2017). *Freud – An intellectual biography*. Cambridge: Cambridge University Press.

# Part I
# Process and outcome

# 1 Trajectory of change in the individual and the diagnostic group

## Transference-focused psychotherapy (TFP) and the treatment of personality pathology

*John F. Clarkin, Nicole Cain and Eve Caligor*

## Introduction

The goal of psychotherapy is to provide a relationship between therapist and patient that leads to change in the patient toward symptom reduction, positive change in difficulties in living, and an increase in quality of life. The theme of this book is to focus on the process of patient change with two perspectives in mind: the perspective of the clinical process between the therapist and patient (Caligor et al., 2018), and a second perspective of capturing the process and outcome of change empirically with the tools of research that provide a source of information independent of the therapist-patient pair (Lutz et al., 2021).

This chapter is focused on the process of the clinical and empirical development of an individual psychodynamic psychotherapy for personality disorder called transference-focused psychotherapy (TFP; Caligor et al., 2018; Yeomans et al., 2015). Individuals with personality disorder have a central difficulty in relating to others, and yet cooperating productively with a therapist is essential for effective psychotherapy (American Psychiatric Association, 2013). This seeming paradox and challenge calls for attention to the evolving relationship between patient and therapist that is the focus of TFP. We illustrate our approach to the empirical development of TFP that provides information not only about changes in the patients as a group, such as done in the typical randomized clinical trial (RCT), but also in-depth information about the trajectory of change in the individual patient by use of special statistical procedures. A single clinical case is used in this chapter to compare individual with group change in TFP. Our approach to tracking the individual patient as well as the group sharing the same diagnosis is consistent with the developing interest in personalized approaches to psychotherapy research and precision medicine (Wright & Woods, 2020). Finally, the process and yield of our clinical and empirical approach can be compared to the typical psychoanalytic case study.

DOI: 10.4324/9781032651934-3

## Aspects of patient change

Therapists and psychotherapy researchers are in pursuit of specifying change that is brought about by psychotherapy. Patient "change" is a global concept that encompasses numerous elements involved in the process that need elaboration. A first question is: What changes? Much of psychotherapy research is focused on symptom change. Do the symptoms that patients present on coming to therapy change in a positive direction during and following psychotherapy? From a more clinical perspective, patients and therapists look for change in symptoms that are troubling the patient but also focus on broader aspects of change that lead to a more satisfying life for the patient, e.g., more satisfying relationships with others.

A further question is: What is the rate of change? How long does it take for change to occur? This is a question of interest not only to the patient but also to insurers and public officials that provide resources for mental health programs. A related question is: What is the sequence of change? For example, does the relationship between the patient and therapist change toward a positive and cooperative manner before symptoms begin to change? Does change in the potential conflicts that surface between patient and therapist change before similar changes in the patients' relationship with those in his/her environment? A further question is about the durability of change: Does the change that occurs during the therapeutic process remain after treatment ends? Or, in fact, does the change that was initiated during treatment not only endure but also accelerates?

A question of intense interest to both therapists and researchers is: What patient characteristics that are revealed during the pre-treatment assessment process predict change from the intervention? What is this patient's prognosis for change? In the psychotherapy research language, what are the patient moderators of change? Finally, a question of intense interest in the clinical and research communities is: What transpires between patient and therapist (Crits-Christoph & Gibbons, 2021) that leads to change? In other words, what are the mechanisms of change? With clear knowledge about the essential mechanisms of change, the field of psychotherapy can refine therapist training and supervision, and result in more efficient and effective interventions. The intense debates between the relative merits of different approaches to psychotherapy (e.g., cognitive behavior therapy and psychodynamic therapy) can be approached with more precision and perspective with knowledge of the mechanisms of change.

### Transference-focused psychotherapy (TFP) and patient change

Otto F. Kernberg and colleagues at the Personality Disorders Institute of the New York Presbyterian Hospital—Cornell and Columbia Medical Centers have developed an object relations based psychodynamic psychotherapy for patients with borderline personality disorder (BPD; Yeomans et al., 2015).

Following empirical assessment for the impact of TFP on patients with BPD (Clarkin et al., 2001; Clarkin et al., 2007; Doering et al., 2010), the scope of TFP has been expanded and applied as a transdiagnostic treatment for patients with a full range of severity of personality pathology (Caligor et al., 2018; Clarkin et al., 2022). As described by DSM-5 alternative model (AMPD) (American Psychiatric Association, 2013) and ICD-11 (World Health Organization, 2021) the essence of all personality disorder is significant disruptions in self-functioning and it impact on functioning with others.

## Origins of TFP in psychoanalysis

Kernberg (American Psychiatric Association, 2013) has proposed that the essential techniques of psychoanalysis are as follows: (1) the use of free association as the basic task of the patient, (2) interpretation, (3) transference analysis, (4) technical neutrality, and (5) utilization of countertransference. TFP is based on these same techniques, but they are employed with significant modification to fit the needs and capacities of personality disordered patients with varying levels of personality organization and compromised identity formation.

In contrast to psychoanalysis, TFP is a structured treatment with its own methods of exploration. TFP was constructed with psychoanalytic understanding of individuals in mind, but with a focus on the specific deficits in patients with mild and moderate-to-severe personality pathology. The traditional approach to psychodynamic treatment was modified to meet the needs of this specific patient group. This orientation led us to articulate aspects of dynamic treatment that could address and cope with the identity diffusion, emotional dysregulation, impulsivity, and the interpersonal difficulties that disrupt work and intimate relations so characteristic of personality disordered patients. TFP is focused on the biased and distorted internal representations of self and others that are related to the external, behavioral manifestations of personality disorder, i.e., the disruptions in relations with others that interfere with normal functioning in the domains of work and interpersonal functioning, spanning friendships to intimate relations. This approach to adapting the psychoanalytic treatment strategies and techniques to the personality disordered group of individuals led to the generation of a treatment manual describing a principle-driven treatment that could manage the clinical challenges presented by this patient population making use of treatment structure, sequence of clarification leading to interpretation, and focus on both the internal representations of self and others and how these representations are manifested in troubling behavior in love and work (Caligor et al., 2018).

## Essential elements of TFP

Object relations theory (Kernberg, 1984) posits the potent effect of mental representations of self and others on self-functioning and functioning in relations with others. Personality pathology involves mental representations that are biased toward a negative view of self and others infused with polarized and intense, extreme emotions of anger and need.

TFP provides the clinician with a treatment for patients with personality disorder with three crucial ingredients: (1) an approach to personality pathology based upon a detailed articulation of personality organization; (2) a clinical assessment approach that enables the clinician to focus the treatment, make a prognosis, and predict areas of treatment focus and potential difficulties given the severity level of the patient; and (3) a principle-driven treatment that has been described in detail for instruction and application (Caligor et al., 2018).

## Patient assessment and contracting

The assessment of personality pathology to set the parameters for treatment with TFP is focused not only on the DSM (American Psychiatric Association, 2013) and ICD standards for diagnosis but also more centrally on the level of personality organization (see Table 1.1; Caligor et al., 2021). The treatment of personality pathology is heavily influenced by the level of personality organization which is the powerful context in which the symptoms and daily functioning occur. The level of personality organization provides preliminary information on the goals of treatment, prognosis, the need for various level of treatment structure, and foci of intervention (Table 1.2).

TFP begins with a thorough clinical assessment to arrive at a DSM diagnosis and a structural diagnosis based on object relations theory. TFP is goal oriented toward not only symptom change but also change in the personality organization that relates to improvement in work/professional life and friendships/intimate relations. During clinical assessment, the patient is asked to reflect upon and clarify his/her treatment goals. At the completion of the assessment, a verbal treatment contract is introduced in which patient and therapist agree on the conditions for attendance and therapy participation that are essential for the treatment to take place.

## Principle TFP intervention strategies and techniques

The focus of TFP treatment exploration is on the patient's present experience rather than the past. The therapist's attention is on both the patient's transference patterns and also on the patient's dominant object relations with current extra-therapy relationships. The TFP therapist balances attention to in-session material with remaining alert to the patient's activity in work and friendships/intimate relations in daily life. The therapist's stance is one of technical neutrality. Interpretation of the patient's dominant object relations as manifested to individuals in the patients' current life and the therapist is the focus of intervention. The process of interpretation flows from identification of the dominant object relations to interpretation from surface to depth (Clarkin et al., 2022).

Table 1.1 Assessment of Levels of Personality Organization

| | Neurotic Organization | High Borderline Organization | Mid-Borderline Organization | Low Borderline Organization |
|---|---|---|---|---|
| STIPO-R level of personality organization | Mature identity formation; some rigidity in functioning | Identity diffusion | Identity diffusion; self-destructive behavior | Identity diffusion; aggression and compromised moral functioning |
| Level of personality functioning in DSM-5, alternative model of personality functioning | Level 1 | Level 2 | Level 3 | Level 4 |
| Typical personality disorder diagnosis/constellation | Obsessive compulsive; depressive; hysterical | Dependent; histrionic; avoidant; narcissistic | Narcissistic; borderline; paranoid; schizoid | Narcissistic, borderline and paranoid with antisocial features; antisocial |
| Nature of self/other functioning | Integrated, realistic and continuous experience of self in relation to others; relationships characterized by mutuality. Rigid functioning in areas of conflict | Somewhat superficial and/or polarized experience of self in relation to others; some capacity for dependency but with conflict | Superficial, extreme, polarized, unstable sense of self in relation to others with gross distortions; need-fulfilling relationships | Extreme, highly polarized and chaotic sense of self in relation to others with gross distortion; exploitative relationships |

Table 1.2 Treatment planning for levels of personality organization

| | Neurotic organization | High borderline organization | Mid-borderline organization | Low borderline organization |
|---|---|---|---|---|
| Prognosis for treatment | Excellent | Good | Fair | Guarded |
| Objectives of treatment | Increase flexible functioning in areas of conflict | Greater depth and stability in experience of self and others | Resolution of destructive behavior; greater depth in experience of self and others | Behavior control; modulation of aggression |
| Structuring (contract setting) of the treatment | Less need for structured contract | Explicitly agreed upon treatment contract | Carefully constructed treatment contract is essential | Contracting must be extensive; focus on secondary gain and safety of patient and therapist |
| Transference process | Develops gradually and is affectively well-modulated. Realistic quality and relative stability over time | Early idealized transferences can keep paranoid object relations out of treatment | Develops rapidly, is affectively charged and extreme. Confusing and chaotic quality with role reversals and abrupt shifts. Early transferences predominantly paranoid | Affectively charged; predominantly paranoid |
| Countertransference | Relatively well integrated in form of thoughts or associations; therapists affected in subtle and socially appropriate ways which may be almost imperceptible at first | Therapist feels less controlled and has more inner space to reflect than with mid/low BPO | Therapist feels controlled and driven to action; can be extremely uncomfortable, difficult to contain, experienced as imposed on | Therapist feels controlled and driven to action; extremely uncomfortable |

## Mechanisms of change in TFP

Patients treated in TFP are significantly more likely to move from an in-secure to a secure attachment style and increase the capacity for reflective functioning (RF) after one year of treatment, as compared to the other therapies (Buchheim et al., 2017; Fischer-Kern et al., 2015; Levy et al., 2006b). The finding that TFP is associated with increases in RF leads to the question of how this is accomplished in the therapeutic process.

In a process study comparing different treatment approaches (Kivity et al., 2019), adherence to prototypical TFP and mentalizing-enhancing interventions was highest in TFP therapists, relative to supportive psychodynamic therapy (SPT) and dialectical behavior therapy (DBT; Linehan, 2018). Higher adherence to TFP principles predicted larger reduction in verbal assault and increase in RF only in TFP, and this finding supports the TFP model of change. In a second process study, therapy sessions were segmented to therapist and patient talk-turns (Kivity et al., 2021), which were rated for bids by the therapist for patients to reflect upon their mental state (i.e., bids for RF) and acoustically coded for arousal. Across three treatments (TFP, DBT, SPT), therapist bids for reflection were twice as common in TFP as compared to the other two treatments and predicted improved post-treatment RF, which in turn predicted lower emotional arousal. These findings suggest that asking patients to reflect upon their mental states has a down-regulatory effect on patients' arousal during the treatment interaction. We conclude that the capacity for RF may be more central in the process and outcome of TFP than for other treatments for BPD such as DBT and good clinical management.

## Research on change in the individual patient and the diagnostic group

Psychotherapy research has been dominated by the RCT which compares the relative efficacy of two or more therapeutic approaches to patients with the same psychiatric diagnosis. The intent is to identify clearly defined therapeutic approaches to a homogeneous group of patients selected by psychiatric diagnosis to control for extraneous variables and arrive at an answer that identifies the most effective treatment approaches to a homogeneous patient group. This "horse race mentality" has led to identifying the best treatment (which horse won the race) for a specific patient group selected by patient diagnosis.

However, this approach has many limitations that have been documented elsewhere, including the extensive heterogeneity of patients who fit into a specific personality disorder category such as BPD. Not only does the diagnostic process of assigning the diagnosis of BPD with any combination of five to nine criteria lead to the identification of a very heterogeneous group but also the so-called "co-morbid" personality disorder conditions (e.g., co-morbid narcissistic and antisocial personality disorder) complicate the assessment and the subsequent treatment.

Our empirical approach has included use of the RCT design, but its limitations have led us to utilize a research approach that features the trajectory of change captured with multiple data points across time for both the individual patient and the diagnostic group in treatment. Thus, we can capture the nature of change across time in both the individual and the group of patients sharing the same diagnosis.

The need to adapt therapeutic intervention by patient characteristics in addition to diagnosis has been referred to as personalized treatment approaches (Cohen et al., 2021). TFP as applied to those with personality disorder is personalized at many points in the treatment process. As described later in this chapter, during the assessment process the level of personality organization determines the degree of structure that must be introduced into the treatment to enable productive therapeutic process. We have generated empirical data to suggest that BPD patients with a full range of pre-treatment RF are suited for TFP, whereas those with relatively high RF respond to DBT (Keefe et al., 2023). Probably, the most personalized aspect of TFP is the identification of the dominant object relations that are unique to each individual patient. With a growing conceptualization of the dominant object relations dyads in the patients' life, the TFP therapist can formulate specific interventions to further patient reflection and change in both behavior and attitudes toward others in their lives.

### Change in the individual patient: a case illustration

As an illustration of our clinical and empirical approach, consider the treatment of a 30-year-old Asian female with the personality disorder diagnosis of BPD. The case provides an opportunity to explicate two features of our approach: (1) the various aspects of change that we have described before (i.e., changes in symptoms, changes beyond symptoms, the speed of change, the sequence of changes), and (2) attention to both the individual patient and the treatment of the entire class of personality disordered patients. The case demonstrates how TFP is delivered to patients in a transdiagnostic manner and how the principles of TFP are applied in the individual case.

### Assessment and case formulation

This 30-year-old single female of Asian descent presented for treatment in the immediate turmoil of having left an intense sadomasochistic relationship of two years with a male live-in partner. She is a college graduate and works in computer applications. Her stated goal for treatment was to improve in her relationships and find a new intimate male companion.

A primary aim in the initial assessment with TFP is to evaluate the level of personality organization as that is central to the nature of the therapeutic relationship, likely issues to arise in the treatment process, and overall prognosis for change. On the STIPO-R the patient (see Table 1.1) had a level of 4 (with 5 being the most severe in a 1 to 5 scale) in Identity and Object Relations and a level 4.5 in Aggression with a slightly better score of 3 on Moral Values. In the perspective of object relations theory, the patient has a low-level borderline personality organization with severe disturbance in identity and quality of object relations, marked self-aggression and aggression toward others, and moderate disturbance in moral functioning.

On more traditional semi-structured interviews for diagnosis, this patient met criteria for BPD and narcissistic personality disorder. She also met criteria for symptom disorders including persistent depressive disorder and social anxiety disorder. Her therapist also provided ratings using the PDM-2 (Lingiardi & McWilliams, 2017) diagnostic system, indicating that she met criteria for narcissistic personality syndrome (vulnerable and malignant subtypes) with a severe level of impairment. This diagnostic impression was confirmed by her self-report scores on the Pathological Narcissism Inventory (Pincus et al., 2009) that were over two SDs above the mean compared to psychotherapy outpatients and her elevated self-report scores on the scales that comprise the malignant narcissism index (Lenzenweger et al., 2018). Finally, using the severity ratings of personality disorder in AMPD of DSM-5 and ICD-11, this patient is at the most severe end.

### TFP is a structured and goal-oriented treatment

Following initial clinical assessment, the TFP therapist describes the treatment contract, the verbal agreement between therapist and patient on the conditions for the therapy to proceed and could succeed. This patient readily agreed to the terms (e.g., present on time for two sessions per week, free association in sessions) of TFP. Throughout the treatment, the patient was present for all sessions in a timely fashion. She complied with the requirement for free association and was quite fluent in her communication of thoughts, feelings, and behavior and her intense involvement with the therapist.

The patient's goal for treatment as stated in the initial assessment process was finding a new boyfriend. The patient's goal was congruent with the TFP therapist's goal of structural change (i.e., identity consolidation, reduced aggression, enhanced moral functioning) in the service of work functioning and functioning in intimate relations.

### TFP: alliance and transference/countertransference

The therapeutic alliance between patient and therapist is traditionally defined in psychotherapy research as congruence between the two participants in terms of therapy goals, treatment methods, and the bond between them.

The construct of therapeutic alliance is related to and partially overlapping with the psychoanalytic concepts of transference and countertransference.

From the very beginning of the treatment, this patient developed an intense connection to the therapist. She readily reported fantasies of sexual and aggressive content involving the patient and the therapist, and, at times, with the therapist and his wife. The dominant object relationship theme was one in which the therapist was fulfilled and superior and the patient was left out, discarded, and destroyed. By around the twelfth month of treatment the patient revealed that she was stalking the therapist on the internet, discovering minute details about the therapist and his wife. Upon the advice of the supervisory group, the therapist told the patient that this intense pursuit of him on the internet must stop or the treatment could not continue. The patient complied, and this structuring of the treatment was followed by the patient's reflection on the possibility of friendships filled with affection rather than aggression. She developed a platonic relationship with a gay man, and the transference with the therapist became slightly erotic without overwhelming aggression.

## Trajectory of domains of change

The case provides an example of our approach to the multiple aspects of change that have been detailed previously in this chapter.

### Changes in the overt content of sessions

A major change in this patient's treatment was advancing from intense fantasies and preoccupation of a sadomasochist relationship with the therapist during the first 14 to 15 months of treatment to a final stage of beginning to imagine an intimate relationship with a man that was affectionate without sadomasochistic intrusion. This patient came to treatment just following the breakup of an intense sadomasochistic relationship. During 18 months of TFP she became intensely attached to the therapist and contained her reflection about relationships without engaging in such relationships during the whole treatment time. At 14 months, she began engaging in extra-therapy friendships and developed a platonic relationship with an Asian man.

### Changes in symptoms, love and work

The patient had 11 previous suicide attempts, and there were none during the treatment period. She worked consistently at her job during the entire treatment. The patient engaged in intense, detailed fantasies of sex and aggression involving the therapist and his wife during the first 14 months of treatment, and this gradually changed to thoughts that she might be able to form an intimate relationship without violence. By the end of the treatment she was examining dating apps.

### Changes in the transference and countertransference

This woman began treatment with a dominant paranoid transference with free associations of mutual aggression and destruction between her and the therapist. By nine months into the treatment, the therapist reported an erotic transference, and by 12 months into treatment a depressive transference.

The therapist was initially alarmed and somewhat frightened by the patient's free associations of sadomasochistic relationships involving the therapist and his spouse. By midway into the treatment the therapist became aware that the patient was searching the internet for intimate details about the therapist and his wife. He was alarmed and asked his consulting colleagues how to deal with this development. Upon their counsel, the therapist informed the patient that the detailed stalking of him on the internet must cease for the treatment to continue. The patient complied with the treatment requirement.

### Changes in the research data

The research data obtained over the duration of the treatment clearly indicate that the patient made important therapeutic gains in her life. Symptoms, especially anger and depression, decreased. Her moral functioning improved and her narcissistic symptoms were less severe. While intensely involved in the relationship with the TFP therapist, she abstained from sadistic intimate relations, and developed satisfying friendships with growing fantasies of intimate relations without sadomasochistic elements.

We use ecological momentary assessment with great success in our research (Meehan et al., in press). By repeatedly asking patients to rate themselves and others in their daily life using smartphone technology at different timepoints in treatment, we can begin to track important shifts in self-other representations. In this case, the patient's perceptions of others in her daily life evolved from rigid, extreme, and mostly negative to much more nuanced. Her capacity to view others as being warm, friendly, and more benign, particularly around themes of dominance and control, improved over the course of treatment. She also began to view herself in more nuanced ways in relation to other people, viewing herself as more capable of warmth and affiliation as treatment progressed.

However, a major question is what are the aspects of TFP that led to the change? What are the actions of the therapist in relationship to the patient that led to change? Our hypothesis is that the TFP therapists' focus on the patients' dominant object relations during treatment leads to a growing ability on the part of the patient to put momentary affect arousal stimulated by conflicted interpersonal interactions into a more benign and broader contextual understanding of self and others. This therapist action and patient re-action is at the essence of mechanisms of change in TFP (Levy, Clarkin, et al., 2006a).

## Comparison of this case with group change

This unique case of the 30-year-old Asian female can be compared to the general trajectory of change for personality disordered patients in TFP. It is most informative to compare the domains and rate of change in this case of a low-level borderline personality organization patient with patient at neurotic, high and moderate levels of personality organization (see Caligor et al., 2018).

It is often the case that a BPD patient will begin treatment in the emotional turmoil following the breakup of a romantic relationship. Some patients come to treatment without romantic involvements, some with short-term sexual contacts only, and some with intense emotional relations during their recent past. In reference to our case study, this patient had the capacity for an intense relationship albeit with a sadomasochistic theme.

It typically takes several months in TFP for the reduction of behavior that interferes with treatment such as missing sessions and not free associating with honesty. This patient while coming faithfully to all sessions on time, began to stalk the therapist on the internet and accumulating detailed information about the therapist and his wife. This stalking behavior is unusual and can be seen as a desperate attempt to both merge with the other but at the same time to attack and destroy the other.

We have found that BPD patients vary tremendously in their expression of attention to and preoccupation with their relationship with the therapist. The patient under discussion was unusual in her intense preoccupation with the therapist from the beginning of treatment. Whereas her attendance at therapy sessions and involvement in treatment were strengths, her intense preoccupation with the therapist and need to almost fuse with him was intensely regressive, frightening to the therapist, and filled with both need and violence.

In previous research, we (Lenzenweger et al., 2018) have found that patients with BPD and malignant narcissism change more slowly than BPD patients without such conditions. The case of this 30-year-old female is consistent with that finding and provides some detail as to how the more complex change in time might occur.

## Summary and conclusions

Psychoanalytic colleagues have made three important criticisms of our approach to the clinical and empirical development of a treatment for personality pathology that deserve a response. First, psychotherapy research is guided by DSM diagnoses and the diagnoses do not capture important dynamics of the individual patient that emerge in the treatment. We agree that the DSM diagnoses, including those on the personality disorders, have serious shortcomings. However, recent changes in the DSM and ICD-11 approach to the diagnosis of personality disorder emphasize difficulties in relating to others with severity ratings that are most helpful for treatment planning. Second, it is pointed out by our critics that treatment manuals stifle the creativity and perceptiveness of the trained therapist. On the contrary, our experience is that even trained analytic therapists are confused and hesitant with severely disturbed personality disorder patients who confront the therapist with their aggressive devaluation of the therapist and treatment. Our manual is principle driven which provides a guide for the therapist without dictating the flow of treatment. Finally, our psychoanalytic colleagues point out that the richness of the individual case gets lost in the research that yields mean scores for the entire group of patients. We take the criticism seriously and utilize statistical approaches that allow us to describe the individual case nested in the group outcome.

The individual case study has been and continues to be a major approach to furthering the understanding of psychopathology and the process of patient change in psychoanalysis. The psychoanalytic case study is an in-depth analysis of a patient in treatment that combines the thoughts, feelings, and reflections of the patient and therapist interventions all seen through the perspective of the therapist. The case illustration presented in this chapter of the TFP treatment of a 30-year-old female with low-level borderline organization can be compared to the typical psychoanalytic case study. The clinical and empirical approach to examining TFP described in this chapter has the advantage of combining multiple perspectives on the single case with the ability to compare the single case to other cases with similar reliably assessed diagnoses.

## References

American Psychiatric Association. (2013). *Diagnostic and statistical manual of mental disorders* (5th ed.). American Psychiatric Association Publishing.

Buchheim, A., Hörz-Sagstetter, S., Doering, S., Rentrop, M., Schuster, P., Buchheim, P., Pokorny, D., & Fischer-Kern, M. (2017). Change of unresolved attachment in borderline personality disorder. *Psychotherapy and Psychosomatics*, *86*(5), 314–316.

Caligor, E., Clarkin, J. F., & Sowislo, J. F. (2021). Levels of personality organization: Theoretical background and clinical applications. In R. E. Feinstein (Ed.), *Primer on personality disorders* (pp. 33–57). Oxford University Press.

Caligor, E., Kernberg, O. F., Clarkin, J. F., & Yeomans, F. E. (2018). *Psychodynamic therapy for personality pathology: Treating self and interpersonal functioning*. American Psychiatric Association Publishing.

Clarkin, J. F., Caligor, E., & Sowislo, J. F. (2022). Transference-focused psychotherapy for levels of personality pathology severity. In H. Crisp & G. Gabbard (Eds.), *Gabbard's textbook of psychotherapeutic treatments* (2 ed.). American Psychiatric Association Publishing.

Clarkin, J. F., Foelsch, P. A., Levy, K. N., Hull, J. W., Delaney, J. C., & Kernberg, O. F. (2001). The development of a psychodynamic treatment for patients with borderline personality disorder: A preliminary study of behavioral change. *Journal of Personality Disorders*, *15*(6), 487–495.

Clarkin, J. F., Levy, K. N., Lenzenweger, M. F., & Kernberg, O. F. (2007). Evaluating three treatments for borderline personality disorder: A multiwave study. *American Journal of Psychiatry*, 164(6), 922–928.

Cohen, Z. D., Delgadillo, J., & DeRubeis, R. J. (2021). Personalized treatment approaches. In M. Barkham, W. Lutz, & L. Castonguay (Eds.), *Bergin and Garfield's handbook of psychotherapy and behavior change. 50th anniversary edition* (pp. 673–703). John Wiley & Sons.

Crits-Christoph, P., & Gibbons, M. B. C. (2021). Personalized treatment approaches. In M. Barkham, W. Lutz, & L. Castonguay (Eds.), *Bergin and Garfield's handbook of psychotherapy and behavior change. 50th anniversary edition* (pp. 298–340). John Wiley & Sons.

Doering, S., Horz, S., Rentrop, M., Fischer-Kern, M., Schuster, P., Benecke, C., Buchheim, A., Martius, P., & Buchheim, P. (2010). Transference-focused psychotherapy versus treatment by community psychotherapists for borderline personality disorder: Randomised controlled trial. *British Journal of Psychiatry*, 196(5), 389–395.

Fischer-Kern, M., Doering, S., Taubner, S., Hörz, S., Zimmermann, J., Rentrop, M., Schuster, P., Buchheim, P., & Buchheim, A. (2015). Transference-focused psychotherapy for borderline personality disorder: Change in reflective function. *The British Journal of Psychiatry*, 207(2), 173–174.

Keefe, J. R., Levy, K. N., Sowislo, J. F., Diamond, D., Doering, S., Hörz-Sagstetter, S., Buchheim, A., Fischer-Kern, M., & Clarkin, J. F. (2023). Reflective functioning and its potential to moderate the efficacy of manualized psychodynamic therapies versus other treatments for borderline personality disorder. *Journal of Consulting and Clinical psychology*, 91, 50–56.

Kernberg, O. F. (1984). *Severe personality disorders: Psychotherapeutic strategies*. Yale University Press.

Kivity, Y., Levy, K. N., Kelly, K. M., & Clarkin, J. F. (2021). In-session reflective functioning in psychotherapies for borderline personality disorder: The emotion regulatory role of reflective functioning. *Journal of Consulting and Clinical psychology*, 89(9), 751.

Kivity, Y., Levy, K. N., Wasserman, R. H., Beeney, J. E., Meehan, K. B., & Clarkin, J. F. (2019). Conformity to prototypical therapeutic principles and its relation with change in reflective functioning in three treatments for borderline personality disorder. *Journal of Consulting and Clinical psychology*, 87(11), 975.

Lenzenweger, M. F., Clarkin, J. F., Caligor, E., Cain, N. M., & Kernberg, O. F. (2018). Malignant narcissism in relation to clinical change in borderline personality disorder: An exploratory study. *Psychopathology*, 51(5), 318–325.

Levy, K. N., Clarkin, J. F., Yeomans, F. E., Scott, L. N., Wasserman, R. H., & Kernberg, O. F. (2006a). The mechanisms of change in the treatment of borderline personality disorder with transference focused psychotherapy. *Journal of Clinical Psychology*, 62(4), 481–501.

Levy, K. N., Meehan, K. B., Kelly, K. M., Reynoso, J. S., Weber, M., Clarkin, J. F., & Kernberg, O. F. (2006b). Change in attachment patterns and reflective function in a randomized control trial of transference-focused psychotherapy for borderline personality disorder. *Journal of Consulting and Clinical Psychology*, 74(6), 1027.

Linehan, M. M. (2018). *Cognitive-behavioral treatment of borderline personality disorder*. Guilford Publications.

Lingiardi, V., & McWilliams, N. (2017). *Psychodynamic diagnostic manual: PDM-2*. Guilford Publications.

Lutz, W., de Jong, K., Rubel, J. A., & Delgadillo, J. (2021). Measuring, predicting, and tracking change in psychotherapy. In M. Barkham, W. Lutz, & L. Castonguay (Eds.), *Bergin and Garfield's handbook of psychotherapy and behavior change. 50th anniversary edition* (pp. 89–133). John Wiley & Sons.

Meehan, K. B., Cain, N. M., Roche, M. J., Sowislo, J. F., Fertuck, E. A., & Clarkin, J. F. (in press). Evaluating change in transference and interpersonal functioning in the treatment of borderline personality disorder: A single-case study using ecological momentary assessment. *Journal of Personality Disorders, 37*(5), 490–507.

Pincus, A. L., Ansell, E. B., Pimentel, C. A., Cain, N. M., Wright, A. G., & Levy, K. N. (2009). Initial construction and validation of the Pathological Narcissism Inventory. *Psychological Assessment, 21*(3), 365.

World Health Organization. (2021). *International classification of diseases, 11th revision (ICD-11)*. World Health Organization.

Wright, G. C., & Woods, W. C. (2020). Personalized models of psychopathology. *Annual Review of Clinical Psychology, 16*(15), 1–15.

Yeomans, F. E., Clarkin, J. F., & Kernberg, O. F. (2015). *Transference-focused psychotherapy for borderline personality disorder: A clinical guide.* American Psychiatric Association Publishing.

# 2 Clinical outcome and process research in the MODE study[1]

## From the psychoanalysis of a young man in emerging adulthood

*Marianne Leuzinger-Bohleber and
Gilles Ambresin*

### Introduction

When the IPA Board in 2017 made the momentous decision that in the future all the different psychoanalytic training models (the Eitingon model, the French model and the Uruguayan model) would be accepted by the IPA, i.e., the training cases with a weekly frequency of three to five sessions would be recognized, it triggered severe anxieties to lose central parts of one´s psychoanalytic identity, well-developed structures and certainties, the good quality of psychoanalytic education and treatment and so on. In the hot, fiercest debates even fundamentalist lines of argument could be observed. Therefore, Mark Solms, the then Chair of the Research Boards of the IPA, proposed to initiate an empirical study on this in order to refer to the Freudian empirical scientific tradition instead of falling prey to fundamentalist wishful thinking or beliefs. The Multilevel Outcome Study of Psychoanalyses of Chronically Depressed Patients with Early Trauma (MODE) study, which we report on in the following, emerged from this institutional context. After two feasibility studies had shown that it was at all possible and practicable to investigate the influence of weekly session frequency on the outcome of psychoanalysis in a large, multicenter, international study, we launched the main study.

The belief outlined in the introduction that psychoanalysis is a science that – unlike religions and Weltanschauungen – is never finished but is in a constant process of critical self-questioning and openness to insights from other disciplines, had many implications for the development of the MODE study design. Already in the LAC depression study, fully aware of the challenging epistemological and methodological problems associated with extraclinical empirical psychotherapy research, psychoanalysis had faced comparison with CBT. It was our conviction that it is crucial for the future of psychoanalysis as a science to counter the prejudice that it is a "faith community" that retreats – in analogy to religious groups – into exclusive communication with like-believers in the psychoanalytic ivory tower, with a large empirical study. In doing so, LAC researchers placed themselves in an often little-known tradition of psychoanalytic empirical researchers,

DOI: 10.4324/9781032651934-4

which had always struggled to hold its own position in the world of medicine and academic science since the very beginnings of psychoanalysis. Thus, it was important that the LAC study could show, according to the strict criteria of evidence-based medicine, that psychoanalysis led to similarly successful statistically significant reductions in depressive symptoms with very high effect sizes, a drastic reduction in the relapse rate in this difficult-to-treat patient group similar to CBT. In addition, the psychoanalytic patients achieved an increased awareness of unconscious fantasies and conflicts (so-called "structural changes"), but needed more sessions for this than CBT, a topic which was and still is discussed in several papers (see, for example, Leuzinger-Bohleber, 2023; Leuzinger-Bohleber & Arnold, 2020, Beutel et al., 2022, and Krakau et al., submitted).

Undeniably, however, the LAC study could not research in detail the many processes that lead to transformations and thus to positive outcomes in psychoanalyses (as, for example, in Mr. P mentioned in the introduction to this volume) with the methodological procedure of the study, because, as we know, there are developmental and change processes "that can only be told and not measured". For this reason, a book with carefully documented, detailed case histories of some psychoanalyses complemented the publications of the results of the LAC study in renowned journals of psychotherapy research (Leuzinger-Bohleber et al., 2020).

## Combining clinical and extraclinical, psychoanalytic and nonpsychoanalytic, process and outcome research strategies in the MODE study

In the LAC study, we applied a broad spectrum of contemporary psychoanalytic research strategies and thereby attempted to meet the current zeitgeist in today's knowledge society without uncritically submitting to it and renouncing the autonomy of psychoanalysis as a scientific discipline. As we will discuss in this chapter, we try to continue this tradition also in the currently ongoing MODE study (Ambresin et al., 2023). In the so-called extraclinical part of our research, we try to meet the requirements of today's randomized, manualized therapy-outcome studies, so that the results of our studies are heard in times of evidence-based medicine. At the same time, we would like to illustrate in this paper that we are also advancing the so-called *Clinical Research of Psychoanalysis* within the MODE study. In the following section of our joint chapters, this kind of clinical psychoanalytic research is presented – as kind of an exemplary case. One finding of the MODE study that was unexpected to us, namely that patients with complete developmental arrest in so-called emerging adulthood can probably be best treated in a high-frequency setting. In the following chapter, we will take up clinical observations of the individual case of Mr. X, namely, that this patient's dreams changed systematically over the course of 15 months of psychoanalysis which is considered as an important indicator of transformations in the patient's inner object world. The chapter will discuss how important finding of clinical psychoanalytic research can be connected in a meaningful and fruitful way with extraclinical researching of the change of dream contents.

## Case illustration: "caught in the poisoned web, I cannot escape the greedy sucking spider…" (Mr. X)[2]

Of course, I (M. Leuzinger-Bohleber) cannot summarize this psychoanalysis in detail here. I would like to try to give at least an impression, on the basis of a few selected sequences of the treatment and above all on the basis of a few dreams, that during the relatively short psychoanalysis, which lasted 15 months, an astonishingly intensive psychoanalytical process developed for me.

### First session

When I pick up Mr. X at the door of my office, he measures me sharply and critically for a very short moment and then avoids eye contact. He seems inhibited and extremely withdrawn into himself. "He doesn't feel at home in his body…" is my first association.

In the first assessment interviews, he speaks in a low voice, often hardly understandable for me. Nevertheless, an emotional contact develops between us. He suffers from severe depression and suicidal thoughts and does not see any perspective for himself and his future. He broke up his pharmacology studies and made a serious suicidal attempt. He sought help from a psychiatrist who prescribed medication but strongly recommended that he start psychotherapy.

### Some biographical information

The 25-year-old patient is the first son of a professor of psychopharmacology and a manager of a big, international bank. He has a younger sister (−2 years). The mother was an illegitimate child of a cleaning woman. The natural father refuses contact with her to this day. The father comes from a traumatized family of academics who fled the former communist Germany in 1960. Working as banker, he was often absent.

It becomes more and more clear in the course of psychoanalysis, that the patient was severely emotionally neglected during his first years. His mother probably suffered from a severe postpartum depression and a lack of empathy for the needs of her baby. With a strange affect, she told her friends, for example, how "sweet" the baby reacted when she spread mustard on her nipples in the 3rd month of life in order to wean him (abruptly). The patient appears to have experienced too few reliable and lasting relationships to develop sustaining affect and drive regulation as well as stable self and object representations.

Possibly, the early relationship with the primary objects was strained by the transgenerational transmission of traumatization related to pregnancy and birth. The patient describes that his relationship with both parents was characterized by high-performance expectations, little emotional continuity and warmth and frequent ruptures and separations.

Therefore, the relationship with the grandfather with whom he felt safe and loved had an important compensatory function. The loss of this good internal and external object, when the grandfather died, intensified the depression of Mr. X in adolescence. After six months of psychoanalysis the patient remembered suddenly that he was forced to sleep in the bed of his grandmother after the death of her husband in order to console her – a highly irritating experience for him at the beginning of puberty. During these months he gained a lot of weight. Even in high school, he seems to have lived in relative isolation and seclusion. Nearly until the end of the first year of psychoanalysis, he lived in his parents' home.

### The psychoanalysis

We started the three-session treatment some months after the assessment interviews, because we had to wait for the evaluation by the insurance company.

The patient resumes his studies maybe as a first result of the assessment interviews. I offer some crisis interventions (one session a week) to stabilize this step and to bridge the weeks until we can start psychoanalysis. The severity of the depression becomes more and more clear during these sessions. The patient lives completely isolated in the house of his parents, is filled with deep resentment and hatred and often sleeps until the afternoon. The contact with him in the sessions is often very strange. I experience the patient often as being in a dissociative state of mind, not really present in the sessions. Sometimes I have the feeling that he does not even seem to know who he really is. I feel reminded of a severe process of identity diffusion or even a threat of a psychotic regression. In other sessions, X´s behavior reminds me of a defiant toddler, withdrawn in himself in great despair. This is often difficult to bear for me, and doubts arise as to whether the patient can be reached psychoanalytically at all. He seems to have withdrawn into a nearly autistic world of his own. The boundaries between self and object, child and adult, men and women, living and dead objects seem to blur. Sometimes, the concept of the anal phallus by Janine Chasseguet-Smirgel (1991) comes to my mind, for example, while listening to the following dream. She had described that the phantasy of the anal phallus may be seen as an unconscious rebellion against psychic differentiation as a developmental step.

> I dreamt of a man who had his own clinic. He was in the garden, looked terrible - very big (all the proportions were not right). He had a terrible disease: the upper body was huge, the lower part of the body was like a cone, with a sinister surface. I cannot describe this at all. Do you know black spiders that carry their children on their backs? This is what this looked like. <u>Spider threads were all around him</u>. I wanted to help the man, but I didn't know how. I also couldn't diagnose what was wrong with him.

Although the dream and the associations frighten me, because they refer to the severely destroyed body image of the patient, I increasingly find an inner contact to the patient while talking about the dream. I have the impression that the patient allows himself to be touched emotionally. This changes again during the next weeks. We are starting the three-session psychoanalysis shortly before the summer break.

*After the vacations*, Mr. X appears in a threatening psychic and psychosomatic state: He has retreated to bed for days with severe suicidal thoughts. He has not done any sports, has eaten a lot and drunk alcohol, so that he has gained several kilos.

The analytic work finally helps him getting out of his severe depressive state in the following weeks. The topic of separation, his enormous unintegrated anger toward the "neglecting object" (the analyst due to the long holidays) are central issues of our psychoanalytic work during these weeks. In connection with these intensive weeks of psychoanalytic work, Mr. X expresses the wish to increase the frequency of weekly sessions to four sessions per week after the fall vacations.

In the first session after the autumn vacations, he reports that he felt much better than during the summer break. He went on an outing with friends. However, it turns out that he got drunk on his birthday because he felt lonely and was envious of the tenderness between his boyfriend and his girlfriend. During the night he woke up from a terrible nightmare:

> You're driving in a car – I'm sitting in the passenger seat, you're wearing a mask, we're silent, we come to a traffic island. That's when I realize something's wrong. There are two lanes. We get in the wrong lane, I get dizzy. Then you turn your head - it's completely distorted on one side - I don't recognize you - I get a fright, can hardly breathe...

The associations lead to his fear of dependence on me, that he will be "disappointed, mixed up and insulted again" if he trusts in me, for example. In my associations I am concerned whether I am "on the wrong track" somewhere. Is something going too fast for the patient? Why does he get dizzy? Is it the reaction to the holiday separation?

Mr. X reports another dream two weeks later. The dream was triggered by a visit to friends who had a baby.

It was a scary dream - I woke up full of disgust....My mother had a baby. I was both the doctor and the father of the child. The child was strangely greenish-yellow. It did not look healthy, may have bled from the mouth. My mother did not want to know about the baby, did not want to breastfeed it. Then I gave it to her to breastfeed. Then the baby got better...

It did not have a name. I suggested Susanna - (Susanna is a nice name, this is what I told my girlfriend at the time, Susanna X sounds quite good...).

We understand the disgust (as a strong emotion) as an attempt to develop boundaries, because "everything is blurred". At some point it occurs to him that the father also appeared in the dream – but sat passively in a chair and said or did nothing... Mr. X himself calls this an Oedipal dream.

It is amazing that you could remember the dream despite all the disgust and shame and tell it to me here....

The theme of the lack of boundaries from the primary objects is the focus of our work in the following sessions. Three weeks later he reports the following dream:

I was with my mother in a kind of barn. She wants to come to my analysis with me to listen. I promised her this at first, but then say this won't work. She says I am raping (or mutilating?) my memories. I get so angry that I grab her by the shoulders. She is light as a feather. I throw her against a table. I take off, not looking back to see if she hurt herself. I decide to go to your place (to his psychoanalysis, MLB).

We talk about his vital aggressive impulses which are necessary to protect him, me and psychoanalysis and draw clear boundaries between him and his real and inner mother. He experiences these impulses as murderous – one reason for his unbearable guilt feelings.

Psychoanalytic session after around 7 months of psychoanalysis.

Mr. X still isn't really able to study systematically and intensively after the Christmas break. Over the weekend, he was promised a second internship in Switzerland[3] (CH).

A:   "Now you even have a choice..."
X:   I had a dream. I was on the phone with a woman from CH. She was the head of the Psychological Institute. During the talk she told me that a man had collapsed next to her. She told me the symptoms. Thanks to

my knowledge from one of my courses at the University I diagnosed a heart attack. Since the woman did not respond, I called the emergency services myself. The person at the phone thought I was belittling him. Then I got so angry that I took care of the man myself over the phone....

   Associations: The day before the dream he had studied diagnostics of heart attack. "This was meaningful, not mindless learning... I now know the exact date of my final University exam ... Maybe I won't come to the analytic sessions 14 days before then...".

A:   "You think it's better not to come to analysis at all for 14 days than maybe look for convenient off – peak hours here (morning or evening)...?"

There is a back and forth about possible dates. I feel him getting angry.

A:   "Do I sense correctly that you are angry with me right now? ..."
X:   "Yes, that's right, I think you wanted to give me a pedagogical hint to get up earlier and then come to you for the session. But I already told you long ago that I didn't think it was a good idea, not even because of the traffic...".
A:   "I'm sure you notice that your voice is much stronger now – the anger at me obviously revives your spirits..."
X:   laughs – "Yes, I guess that's true..."
A:   "And you now dare to directly contradict me, because you seem to have developed enough trust in me that you can show me your anger, knowing that you don´t destroy me when you correct me for being unempathetic."
X:   "You're just not my mother..."
A:   "Indeed – however we have seen here that you sometimes experience me as similarly unempathetic as your mother – but then it is important that we both notice this. After all, this is our joint task here."

We then talk about many of his memories which illustrate that his mother seemed to associate aggression with catastrophes, which stimulated the unconscious conviction of Mr. X. that he could destroy his objects with his aggressive-destructive impulses.[4]

*Some remarks on the course of psychoanalysis until the end of the first year of treatment*

In the next three months, the focus of the psychoanalytic work is on preparing for the difficult final exam at the University. As the dreams described above show, there exists a great danger of a negative therapeutic reaction: The triumph of failing and thus taking revenge on his mother (and me as the analyst) often proves to be very attractive. In order to make him aware of this unconscious seduction of an archaic revenge, I tell him in one session the fable of the scorpion and the frog, which I know through John Steiner (2003). A scorpion asks a frog to carry him on his back across a river. The frog finally agrees, thinking the scorpion will not bite him, otherwise he will perish and die along with him. But the temptation to sting the frog is too great: The scorpion strikes and they both drown in the river. – Mr. X seems to understand the message and keeps coming back to this fable frequently.

In this way, I try to address the archaic aggressive impulses of the patient again and again, also in the transference relationship with me. As is well known: Access to one's aggressive impulses is central to the psychic differentiating processes between self and object, especially in depressed patients, in whom the psychically aggressive impulses, which are necessary for the separation from the object, often are experienced as murderous and destructive and are therefore directed against the self.

Thus, working through the aggressive-destructive impulses and the unconscious fantasies associated with them proved to be central to the psychic transformation processes of Mr. X particularly in sessions around the exams. To mention just one example: Again and again, I have to free myself inwardly from letting the final exam become a "destructive performance test" of psychoanalysis and assure myself that it is ultimately the decision of the patient whether or not he wants to pass the exam. I try to empathize with the unconscious fantasies of the patient, which indeed often have an apocalyptic dimension: the exam – in his fantasies – is indeed a matter of life and death.

The patient passes his exams and begins a demanding internship in an internationally renowned company. He moves out of his parental home and sets up his own apartment for the first time in his life. The most important fantasy is that he can sleep with a girlfriend in the new bed, "far away from his mother's eyes".

We can only mention in the limited space of this paper that these changes in the patient's external reality also had an enormous effect on the transformations in his inner object world. He experiences a lot of recognition and social affection at his new job, which he was able to experience as an enormous narcissistic gratification and supply for his unstable self-regulation. In one session some weeks later, he says:

> It is so good to work, to make the experience that I am well-liked and appreciated by everybody personally and because I really know a lot—this does not correspond to my view of myself at all: I realized that in depth I don´t really know who I am. Sometimes I think I was only playing different social roles until now….

The strengthened feeling of a stable core self and identity facilitates the analytic work on the massive conflicts triggered by the (real) separation from the parents. It becomes clear that he is unconsciously convinced that he will murder his primary object if he detaches from it. On the other hand, this separation process triggers such archaic feelings of guilt, that he has the fantasy that he has to kill himself.

In the transference relationship analogous fantasies emerged: After the summer holidays he forgets the first analytic session:

> Like you, like me.... You haven't been there for me for a long time - now I don't need you either... you did not exist in my mind yesterday....

The therapeutic work on the psychic integration of his aggressive-destructive impulses is often at the center of the analytic sessions during these weeks and is associated with a surge in identity development.

It is especially important in the coming weeks that the separation conflicts and the pathological mourning processes, triggered by the date when he will move to Switzerland, can now be directly observed in the transference relationship and thus become the object of psychoanalytic understanding.

In a session about four weeks before the end of psychoanalysis Mr. X is full of resentment and depressive feelings. He complains about old patients, whom he had to investigate in his research project, who "stink and will die soon anyway". He then sinks into a long silence. I guess that he is absorbed by his unconscious death wishes toward me as an "elderly analyst who should die soon". He finally tells me that he had a binge eating attack yesterday, that he hates his body and generally thinks that everything here in psychoanalysis has been of no use. "Nothing has changed. I feel as miserable as ever... psychoanalysis was just a big expensive shit..." I am flooded with anger, resentment, helplessness and powerlessness as well as by thoughts like

> Maybe the patient is right, maybe the one year of treatment was really too little, couldn't really cut through the knot of stagnation in his development, reach his deep depression...

I try to understand these emotions, to hold and contain them and to control my feelings professionally. However, I am sure that the analysand is aware of my intensive anger.

This dynamic repeats itself in a similar way in the coming sessions and comes to a head to such an extent that after one particularly difficult session, I am afraid that the patient might break off the treatment shortly before its official end.

He comes on time to the next session and begins with the remark:

> I must have hit you very hard in the last session... I thought that this was too much for you and that now you will throw me out of psychoanalysis...

We can draw the parallel with his fantasy mentioned above that he is unconsciously convinced that he will kill his primary objects if he separates from them.

> And you were convinced that I was "throwing you out" here after the session yesterday, that I don´t want anything more to have to do with

you, which, as we now see, becomes understandable because of your murderous fantasies about separations from important persons. Yet you came on time for the session today and had the courage to look with me into these dark abysses of your psyche - this is anything but a given, that takes quite a lot of courage.[5]

After this session, the patient seems to calm down, and we can talk about his feelings concerning the end of psychoanalysis in a more reflective way. I have the impression that I succeeded in a good enough way to understand and emotionally hold the patient's murderous impulses and thus communicate to him, that I – as an analytic object – have survived his attacks and that our inner relationship and bonding are not destroyed. In spite of all my doubts, if psychoanalysis can really be terminated at this point, I finally tell him:

> We have understood together how important it is for you to take the step to go abroad now alone, without any real contact with me, autonomously, but still connected to me inside.

Mr. X himself – in contrast to me – seems to be quite confident in saying good-bye to me. He leaves open the question if he will contact me again.

He gets in touch with me shortly before Christmas (three months after the end of psychoanalysis) and wants to have a few sessions. He tells me that he was doing amazingly well, especially because he was highly esteemed and successful as a young pharmacologist in a research position.

> Of course, I still have a lot ahead of me…. I will contact you if I think this will do me good…

### Short reflection of the clinical case

Mr. X was in a very vulnerable mental and psychosocial state when he was sent to the psychoanalytic treatment by his psychiatrist: His mental development had come to a complete standstill. He had withdrawn into an autistic-like shell, spent his days depressed in bed at his parents' house, had dropped out of his studies and had hardly any social contacts. In the sessions (once a week), bridging the time until the psychoanalysis could start, I had great doubts about being able to reach the patient psychoanalytically at all. Looking back on this psychoanalysis, I have the impression that a high-frequency setting (first three, then four weekly sessions) was necessary to break the patient's developmental blockade: An intensive transference relationship developed, which made it possible to address and work through the patient's aggressive-destructive impulses and fantasies rather directly, already as part of the transference, at an early stage of the treatment. On the basis of impressive dreams, it became apparent how much the boundaries between self and object representations, pregenital and Oedipal fantasies and conflicts, as well as the barriers between generations and genders had merged in the inner object world of the patient. These psychic realities became successively accessible in the psychoanalytic process.

As is well known, such mental differentiation processes always take place simultaneously, in the external world as well as in the transference relationship. These processes could be observed in an impressive way in this psychoanalysis. Encouraged by the analytic work, he dared to postpone his final university examination date against his mother's will, to move out of the parental home and to plan a training stay abroad. These changes in the outside reality had an enormous influence on the psychic and psychosocial situation of the patient, as well as on transformations in his inner object world. One example was mentioned above: Success with passing the exam and leaving home led to new narcissistic gratifications and new social relationships in the outside world, which strengthened his fragile self-esteem, his autonomy and encouraged him to turn to new objects. At the same time, it was essential to work through central unconscious fantasies connected with the separation and identity-finding processes, mobilizing homicidal and suicidal impulses in the transference, probably unconscious sources of Mr. X's severe depressive breakdown. As Winnicott (1971) described it a long time ago: The survival of the object was essential for coping with the archaic aggressive-destructive fantasies and impulses as well as with the immense guilt feelings connected with them.

From a treatment point of view, the handling of the serious conflicts in connection with the separation and individuation processes of Mr. X was particularly demanding. My first association: "He doesn't feel at home in his body..." probably hit the bull's eye: Mr. X's body unconsciously still belonged to the mother and was therefore the object of archaic destructive impulses and fantasies, as well as a deep refusal to renounce infantile longings and desires and to give up the self-image of a "sexless" infant to be nurtured and held. As a result of the traumatogenic pathological object relationship, self-agency, as well as primal trust in a helping, empathic object had collapsed: the flight into a passive "dead" dissociative inner state was part of an unconscious revenge against the depressed, psychologically abusive primary object: A central unconscious fantasy of the patient was that he was *caught in the poisoned web and could not escape the greedy sucking spider anyway*, and therefore turned the passively feared into an active "fact" himself: He transformed himself into an empty, dead shell in which no life could be found anymore. Mr. X also presented an unconscious sadistic triumph, a fantasy of revenge on his objects, since no one managed to really help him and put him out of his misery. It was important to understand not only the regressive quality of these fantasies but also the progressive impulse to gain autonomy and become less dependent on the (primary) objects. Discovering these unconscious fantasies and working through the life-threatening conflicts and impulses in the transference relationship was the prerequisite for breaking through the developmental blockade and re-starting the self- and identity-finding process of emerging adulthood.

The complex treatment-specific problems of psychoanalytic work with late adolescents and patients in emerging adulthood cannot be addressed in detail in this framework. We just have to refer to other papers in which we have discussed these topics (cf. Bohleber, 2010; Bohleber & Leuzinger-Bohleber, 1981; Freud, 1937; Freud, 1965; Lemma, 2010; Leuzinger-Bohleber, 2023). Just a few comments: Peter Blos (1967) spoke decades ago of the symbolic matricide (and patricide) that is unavoidable in connection with the adolescent process of detachment and individuation. This knowledge helped to understand more adequately the extreme intensity of the pa-tient's aggressive-destructive impulses and fantasies in the transference, to open a space for them and to bear and contain them emotionally in concrete analytical sessions. On the other hand, discussions in recent psychoana-lytic literature on adolescence argue that autonomy and dependency are no longer seen as insurmountable opposites: They are always two poles of hu-man relationships. These concepts were helpful, for instance when it came to communicating to Mr. X that ending psychoanalysis was not a question of breaking off the relationship with the analyst completely, but of arrang-ing it according to his own specific (autonomous) wishes in the future and of transforming the inner feelings of dependencies. The interpretative work based on these conceptualizations probably enabled the patient to contact his analyst again three months after the official ending of the psychoanaly-sis (see section below).[6]

However, as I mentioned above, I was very worried whether the pa-tient's omnipotent defenses would collapse after the short psychoanaly-sis ended and whether the patient would experience another severe depressive breakdown during his stay abroad. I was therefore relieved to hear from the patient that this was not the case in the first few weeks after the termination. But only the coming years will show whether the patient can integrate his omnipotence fantasies into a sustaining narcissistic self-regulation. Therefore, inwardly I very much agree with the patient who said in the follow-up interview: "Of course, I still have a lot ahead of me...."

## Discussion

In this presentation, some first clinical observations with young adults in the frame of the ongoing MODE Study were presented and illustrated with an extensive case example. Mr. X has many characteristics that also apply to "normal" young people during emerging adulthood, including the insta-bility, the strong self-focus/narcissistic feature, the high rate of depression, the delay in identity development and the strong dependency on his par-ents, particularly his mother (see Arnett, 2000, 2015; Leuzinger-Bohleber, 2023; Seiffge-Krenke & Weitkamp, 2020). However, his psychic develop-ment had completely collapsed and ended in a state of severe depression, an extreme withdrawal which would have been difficult to overcome in shorter or less intensive treatments. Hence, the detailed case study wanted to raise the question of whether there is a *specific indication for high-frequency psychoanalysis in patients in emerging adulthood in today's world of globalization and internationalization*. In patients like Mr. X, the separation and individuation process has come to a complete standstill, a standstill that seriously threatens the further life of these patients.

The relatively short psychoanalysis of 15 months, helped Mr. X to resume his collapsed developmental process of emerging adulthood. He regained a certain sense of agency and a basic trust in (new) objects – which is absolutely essential for (traumatized) adolescents and young adults – which he also used in his separation process from the analyst. For him, as for many patients in this developmental phase, it can suddenly be more important to plunge into real life and its (love) relationships than to remain for years in the transference relationship with the analyst.

Of course, the outlined 15 months of analytic work do not correspond to the length of most psychoanalyses in Germany. The average number of sessions in the LAC Depression Study was 254 sessions (see Leuzinger-Bohleber et al., 2019). For Mr. X it was an intensive treatment phase, which the patient may continue abroad or after his return to Germany, if he so wishes. However, by the intensive psychoanalysis he was able to make an important step in the (real and inner) separation from his primary objects and his individuation process.

Similarly unexpected observations have been collected in many of the ongoing psychoanalyses of MODE study. We consider them as a result of clinical psychoanalytic research that we would like to present here for discussion. These observations correspond to a characteristic basic attitude of psychoanalysis which has existed from its beginning on, but that needs to be rediscovered and specified again and again: It seems worthwhile to adapt our psychoanalytic offers to the life cycle of young people in changing specific societal situations. Nowadays, a high-frequency, intensive psychoanalysis, which is open in terms of the length of the treatment and also takes into account the possibility of intensive psychoanalytic work with high weekly intensity but with a limited total duration (in months or years) could be a specific indication for patients in emerging adulthood with a collapsed development. In the best case such offers might prevent pathological developments and the formation of chronic courses of developmental crisis, ending up in chronic depression.

## Notes

1  This large international, multicenter research project, the *Multi-Level Outcome Study of Psychoanalyses of Chronically Depressed Patients with Early Trauma (MODE)*, investigates outcomes of manualized, highly frequent psychoanalytic long-term psychotherapies versus low frequent psychoanalytic long-term psychotherapies for chronic depressed, early traumatized patients with neurobiological, psychological and psychoanalytic. The participating centers of the study are Frankfurt,

Cologne, Leipzig, Giessen, Mainz (Germany), Lausanne (Switzerland) and Los Angeles/San Francisco (USA). The study is supported by the IPA, the ApsaA, the Alfred-Berman-Foundation, the Robert S. Wallerstein Fellowship, the German Psychoanalytic Association (DPV), and the Deutsche Gesellschaft für Psychoanalyse, Psychotherapie, Psychosomatik und Tiefenpsychologie (DGPT).

2   In order to protect the confidentiality, some details of his biography have been actively changed.

3   Because of my accent, the patient knows that I come from Switzerland.

4   This material from the session may illustrate that I followed the patient's associations to the dream and picked up the aggressive impulses and fantasies in the transference. The omnipotence fantasies which were so evident in the manifest dream, and probably served as a defense against the aggressive impulses toward his Swiss psychoanalyst, were not directly addressed at this point with regard to the important function of omnipotent phantasies in emergent adulthood (see below).

5   This last sentence may serve as an example of an interpretation which tries to take account of the extreme narcissistic vulnerability of the patient (see, for example, Gullestad & Killingmo, 2020).

6   In the meantime, after more than a year abroad, the patient contacted the analyst again and asked for a few more analytical sessions.

### References

Arnett, J.J. (2000). Emerging adulthood. A theory of development from the late teens through the twenties. *American Psychologist*, 200, 469–480.

Arnett, J.J. (2015) (Ed). *The Oxford handbook of emerging adulthood*. New York: Oxford University Press.

Ambresin, G., Leuzinger-Bohleber, M.N., Fischmann, T., Axmacher, N., Hattingen, E., Bansal, R., Peterson, B. (2023). The Multi-Level Outcome Study of Psychoanalyses for Chronic Depressed Patients with Early Trauma (MODE). Rationale and Design of an International Mutlicenter Randomized Controlled Trial. Accepted for publication, *BMC Psychiatry*, (2023)23: 844. https://doi.org/10.1186/s12888-023-05287-6.

Beutel, M.E., Krakau, L., Kaufhold, J., Bahrke, U., Grabhorn, A., Hautzinger, M., Fiedler, G., Kallenbach-Kaminski, L., Ernst, M., Rüger, B., Leuzinger-Bohleber, M. (2022). Recovery from chronic depression and structural change: 5-year outcomes after psychoanalytic and cognitiv-behavioural long-term treatments (LAC depression study). *Clinical Psychology & Psychotherapy*, 2022, 1–14. https://doi.org/10.1002/cpp.2793.

Blos, P. (1967). The second individuation process in adolescence. *Psychoanalytic Study of the Child*, 22, 162–87.

Bohleber, W. (2010). *Destructiveness, Intersubjectivity and Trauma: The Identity Crisis of Modern Psychoanalysis*. London: Karnac Books.

Bohleber, W. and Leuzinger, M. (1981). Narzissmus und Adoleszenz. In: Psychoanalytisches Seminar Zürich (Hg.). Die neuen Narzissmustheorien. Zurück ins Paradies? Frankfurt a.M.: Syndikat, 117–131.

Chasseguet-Smirgel, J. (1991). Sadomasochism in the perversions: Some thoughts on the destruction of reality. *Journal of the American Psychoanalytic Association*, 39(2), 399–415.

Freud, S. (1937). Analysis terminable and interminable. S.E. XXIII, 216–57.

Freud, A. (1965). *Normality and Psychopathology in Childhood*. New York: International University Press.

Krakau, L., Ernst, M., Hautzinger, M., Beutel, M., Leuzinger-Bohleber, M. (submitted). *Long-term psychotherapy of chronic depression and early trauma: Differential benefits of psychoanalytic compared to cognitive behavioral treatments.*

Lemma, A. (2010). An order of pure decision: Growing up in a virtual world and the adolescent's experience of being-in-a-body. *Journal of the American Psychoanalytic Association, 58*(4), 691–714.

Leuzinger-Bohleber, M. (2023). „Il fili di ragno lo circondavano" Lánalisi´ad alte frequenza´ è una buona scelta per gli arresti evolutivi nello "stato adulto emergente"? *Rivista di Psicoanalisi*, 2023, LXIX, 2, 1–26.

Leuzinger-Bohleber, M., Arnold, S.E. (2020). Introduction: outcome research and the future of psychoanalysis. In: Leuzinger-Bohleber, M., Solms, M., Arnold, S.E. (eds.). *Outcome Research and the Future of Psychoanalysis. Clinicans and Researchers in Dialogue*. London: Routledge, 1–26.

Leuzinger-Bohleber, M., Donié M, Wichelmann, J., Ambresin, G., Fischmann, T. (2024). Changes in dreams - the development of a dream-transformation scale in psychoanalyses with chronically depressed, early traumatized patients, accepted for publication by the Scandinavian Psychoanalytic Review

Leuzinger-Bohleber, M., Hautzinger, M., Fiedler, G., Keller, W., Bahrke, U., Kallenbach, L., Kaufhold, J., Ernst, M., Negele, A., Schoett, M., Küchenhoff, H., Günther, F., Rüger, B., Beutel, M. (2019). Outcome of psychoanalytic and cognitive-behavioural long-term therapy with chronically depressed patients: a controlled trial with preferential and randomized allocation. *The Canadian Journal of Psychiatry, 64*(1), 47–58.

Leuzinger-Bohleber, M., Solms, M., Arnold, S.E. (eds.) (2020). *Outcome Research and the Future of Psychoanalysis. Clinicans and Researchers in Dialogue*. London. Routledge.

Seiffge-Krenke, I. and Weitkamp, K. (2020). How individual coping, mental health, and parental behavior is related to identity development in emerging adults in seven countries. *Emerging Adulthood 8/5*, 344–360.

Steiner, J. (2003). *Psychic retreats: Pathological organizations in psychotic, neurotic and borderline patients*. Routledge.

Winnicott, D.W. (1971) *Playing and reality*. New York: Basic Books, Inc.

# 3 Changes in dreams – an indicator for transformation processes in psychoanalysis

## Clinical outcome and process research in the MODE study

*Gilles Ambresin and Marianne Leuzinger-Bohleber*

### Introduction

In the last decade, the evaluation of psychotherapies has shifted from a paradigm favouring randomized clinical studies of disorders to studies that explore factors that contribute to changes identified as relevant to clinical practice (Thurin, 2017). Psychoanalytic psychotherapy research is currently facing this challenging task of being able to conduct research that promotes the translation of research findings into clinical practice (Luyten, 2012). After recalling that psychoanalytic research has presented itself as a plural science of the unconscious from the beginning, this chapter will present a conceptual research framework that allows for the articulation of different research modalities. The case study presented in the previous chapter will be used to illustrate the collaboration between the researcher and the clinician that an integrative model of research allows.

### Plurality of research: conceptual framework

#### A bridge between clinical research and empirical research in psychoanalysis

As the case narrative of Leuzinger-Bohleber illustrated in the previous chapter, the research setting in psychoanalysis develops around the analytic session, the site of the encounter between the analyst and the patient. This encounter takes place under the rules of free association and evenly suspended attention, ignoring the manifest content in an attempt to grasp what the patient wishes to convey (Green, 2003). The analyst will then establish relationships between what patients think, feel and are moved by within themselves in order to establish connections between different levels such as affects, bodily states, memory, language and conscious or unconscious fantasies to mention but a few. This listening and formulation activity mobilizes the analyst's latent and explicit theories, while at

DOI: 10.4324/9781032651934-5

the same time, he develops mini-theories, ad hoc, which allow the analyst to be worked on by the clinical material he is confronted with. The second stage, starting with the analyst back at the writing desk for his end-of-session notes or in a perspective of a communication to his peers, calls upon the analyst's analytical concepts which participate in a more or less formal and univocal way in theoretical models shared by the scientific community. This transition from private theories to theoretical models implies an effort to clarify, formulate and/or reformulate psychoanalytic concepts, to better shape the results that emerge from one's research in the clinical setting. By decreasing the elasticity of their concepts, psychoanalytic researchers allow for better communication with peers and will be in a better position to use this new knowledge in future sessions in a kind of feedback loop (Leuzinger-Bohleber, 2015).

This greater conceptual clarity will also provide a bridge to empirical or interdisciplinary research that will complement the traditional clinical debate.

This bridge to empirical research is of interest to psychoanalysis as it was conceived from its beginning as a plural science of the unconscious (Leuzinger-Bohleber, 2018). As Freud wrote in the New Introductory Lessons on Psycho-Analysis psychoanalysis "is a part of science and can adhere to the scientific Weltanschauung" (1933, 181). Freud had shown an interest in experimental studies to support his new psychology. Between 1903 and 1906, the Burghölzli group in Zurich conducted experiments on associations that enabled Bleuler, then director of the Burghölzli, to write that "association is a fundamental phenomenon of psychic activity" in his preface to the results of the Burghölzli research group that included Jung and Riklin. Freud will write to Jung:

> Now that you, Bleuler and to some extent Löwenfeld have won me a hearing among the readers of the scientific literature … the movement in favour of our new ideas will continue irresistibly despite all the efforts of the moribund authorities.
>
> (cited in Makari, 2008, 197)

We can now move forward to examine how contemporary research methods can enable empirical research activity in psychoanalysis.

As presented in the previous chapter, during in-depth clinical discussions of a Multilevel Outcome Study of Psychoanalyses of Chronically Depressed Patients with Early Trauma (MODE) case presentation, a developmental recovery in a young adult with severe developmental blocks (stabilization of the process of autonomy from the parental home and his search for professional and personal identity) was noticed. Clinicians also noticed that the content of the patient's dreams evolved during the high-frequency therapy. To briefly summarize, over time, he presented fewer nightmares, was able to present a more successful resolution of problems as they appeared in the dream, the affective spectrum broadened and he presented more mature object relations. Finally, the dreamer was less often in the position of dream-observer, a position that is considered indicative of the effect of the trauma on participation in the social reality of the dream. From this brief example, it can be noted that a few steps are necessary to "translate" the clinical observations into possible research objects. Here we will introduce five categories of evaluation of the evolution of the dream, each step implying a simplification of the information collected during the clinical encounter. Our summary here of the changes in the dreams says nothing about the richness of the clinical exchanges that took place, but it does indicate how clinician and researcher were able to come to an agreement in attempting to measure the evolution of the dreams. The research communicates its findings in a more abstract way. These steps are critical and can be perilous and require close collaboration between clinician and researcher. Finally, in the context of research, the clinical observations will need to be repeated to support initial insights.

The observation of a detailed clinical case in a randomized clinical trial (RCT) opens clinical and theoretical questions that challenge standard analytical practice. For example, clinicians were able to suggest that if, through high-frequency treatment over a year, this young patient with a near-complete developmental blockage due to chronic depression could be relieved from chronic depressive symptomatology and creatively turn back to age-appropriate developmental tasks, it might suggest that young patients could interrupt the psychotherapeutic process they have begun and possibly continue it later. This approach could allow an initial engagement in care, especially for patients in their 20s and 30s needing frequent treatment, in today's globalized world, where it is often virtually impossible for them to engage in several years of psychoanalysis.

## Case studies in randomized clinical trials

The "Case Studies within Psychotherapy Trials" (CWT) model offers a particularly interesting opportunity to foster close collaboration between clinicians and researchers (see Fishman et al., 2016). CWTs are in-depth clinical case studies of participants in a randomized clinical trial (RCT).

The strength of CWT is that they can be selected and described from the RCT data (Figure 3.1). Fishman and colleagues (2016, ix) argue that the world of "numbers about variables within groups" and the world of "words about patterns within specific individuals" are both of great value in psychotherapy research. We can agree that these two worlds are equally valuable in our field of research. These different perspectives are brought together when an in-depth case study is drawn from an experimental arm of an RCT, as in the example from the MODE study above. Ultimately, the sum of these two perspectives will be greater than their parts. In the brief case presentation in the previous chapter, the empirical and extra-clinical

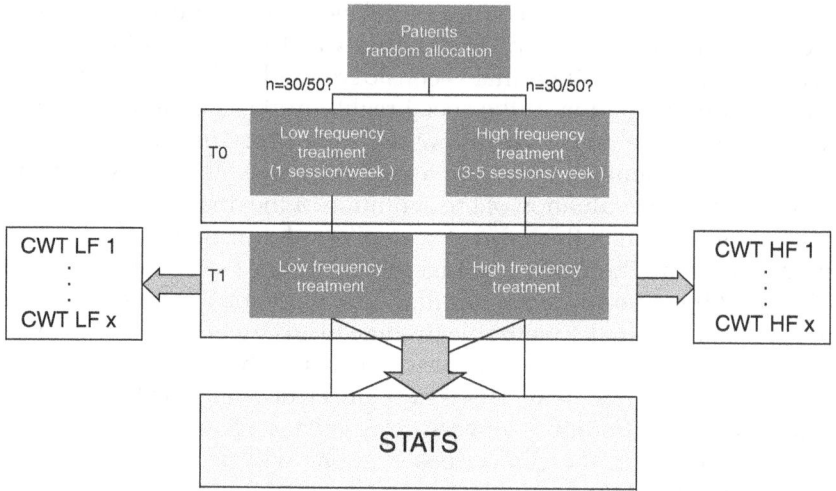

*Figure 3.1* The CWT model.

data of the case could not be presented. Nevertheless, at this stage, the clinical discussion has focused on a case from an RCT and when the results of the neurobiological, psychological and psychoanalytical measures will be available, we will resume the process of exploring the findings with the complementarity of the clinical and extra-clinical perspectives allows.

So, although the case presentation in this paper belongs to the tradition of so-called "case-based learning", we can also consider it a "theory building case study" (Stiles, 2009). In case-based learning, theory is applied to the case. In a research perspective, it is about applying the case to the theory. As such, the detailed clinical observations of the case on the psychoanalytic process offer an opportunity to evaluate and possibly improve the theory.

Much has been written about the use of clinical case reports in psychoanalysis, particularly for patients with chronic depression. Reporting on the development of expert-validated narrative case reports in the LAC study (Leuzinger-Bohleber et al., 2020) that preceded the MODE study, the authors considered this development as "the most important result of the study" (Leuzinger-Bohleber et al., 2016, 10). They went on to write, "These case studies bring psychoanalytic insight into the specific psychodynamics of chronic depression, its complex individual and cultural determinants, and the details of treatment, to the psychoanalytic and non-psychoanalytic community" (Leuzinger-Bohleber et al., 2016, 10). Indeed, case studies are often the most likely way to convey complex experiences to therapists and psychoanalysts and it seems useful to follow the tradition of so-called case-based-learning (cf. Leuzinger-Bohleber & Westenberger-Breuer, 2020; Wallerstein, 1986).

We also know that these in-depth case reports as a scientific method have been challenged by researchers in related research fields. Kächele (2020, 75) listed some criticisms of case reports, such as their anecdotal value, the fact that they lead to inflation of the prevailing theory, that they are not representative of a sample of patients, to name a few. To address these criticisms, attempts have been made to recommend standard methods for the study of case reports that would improve their completeness, clinical relevance, reliability and validity, but with little impact on published psychoanalytic articles (Leuzinger-Bohleber et al., 2020, 251). Our suggestion is that case studies in psychotherapy within RCTs provide an opportunity to resituate them in the context of empirical psychotherapy research, while retaining their heuristic qualities.

From a research perspective, a case study is involved in theory building if it allows researchers to "creatively modify their theories by adding to them (abductively) or altering them to fit the accumulated observations" (Stiles, 2009). Abduction here means creation, refinement and elaboration of theory. "In this way, case observations permeate theories, so that the words of the theory convey the accumulated experience of previous researchers" (Stiles, 2009).

### Transformations in manifest dreams during psychoanalyses: an example for translational research

So far, the detailed case presentation discussed the development of an important transferential relationship and the complex interaction of the patient's personality with his life history, his presenting symptoms, and his present life situation. Developments on the challenges of late adolescence and emerging adulthood presented in the previous chapter together with the clinical observations brought to light challenging questions as regards psychoanalytic technique.

Considering the title of the current volume "Psychoanalytic studies of change. An integrative perspective" aiming at promoting and intensifying the dialogue between psychoanalytical researchers and clinicians, these elements bring to mind the question: "How can we take up the observations reported above formulated from a clinical perspective into questions and methods compatible with clinical and extra-clinical research?"

As mentioned above, the MODE study will explore changes in psychoanalyses as measured with changes in dreams. In clinical practice dream interpretation is "The interpretation of dreams is the royal road to a knowledge of the unconscious activities of the mind" (Freud, 1900, 608) and stays central to psychoanalysis. It is no surprise that psychoanalytic researchers are also interested in dreams as an indicator of the psychoanalytic process as well as an outcome. To analyse dreams from a research perspective, sophisticated methods, such as the Zurich Dream Process Coding System (ZDPCS) have been developed (Fischmann et al., 2021; Moser & von Zeppelin, 1996). The ZDPCS is rather complex and needs specialized training. Our research perspective will refer to another method developed by Leuzinger-Bohleber (1987, 1989). A cross-validation study between the method presented in this chapter and the ZDPCS is currently ongoing.

### *Changes in the manifest dreams in a theory-guided content analysis of five single case studies (dream content analysis by Leuzinger-Bohleber)*

Leuzinger-Bohleber (1987, 1989) compared manifest and latent dreams of the first and last 100 sessions in five psychoanalyses. Systematic changes were found to be significant in aggregated single case studies. In the "successful psychoanalyses" (defined by the analysands, their analysts and independent observers) the following changes in the dreams in the last 100 psychoanalytical sessions were found: (1) the atmosphere of the manifest dream is more frequently positive; (2) more successful problem-solving; (3) broader spectrum of affects (in contrast to the domination of one single affect (most frequently panic) in the dreams of the first 100 sessions; (4) dreamer was in an active position (not in the position of the observer); (5) more intensive and satisfying human relationships; (6) more human subjects, fewer animals. These findings were replicated by Kaechele et al. (2012). Importantly, these studies convincingly show that dream reports can be trusted as a research tool and that they do not represent confabulations or unreliable indications, as has often been suggested.

Following on these findings and within the frame of the MODE study, a group of researchers took up the five categories and worked on their operationalization aiming to obtain a coding system that is reliable and that can be easily taught. We gathered them in a **DRE**ams **A**ssess**M**ent **S**cale for measuring **C**hanges in manifest dreams (DREAMS-C)[1] and named the five categories as:

1 Nightmares;
2 Problem solving;
3 Affective spectrum;
4 Self-agency; and
5 Object relations.

The fifth category will be scored with the SCORS-G (Stein & Slavin-Mulford, 2017) in the future but was not used in this chapter.

> Analysis of the dreams of the case illustration: "Caught in the poisoned web, I cannot escape the greedy sucking spider…" (Mr.X.) with the DREAMS-C.

Using the DREAMS-C, we examined the dreams of Mr X.'s detailed case study focusing on five points: nightmares, problem solving, affective spectrum, self-agency (indicative of dissociation as in trauma, activity of the dreamer in the dream) and maturity of object relations.

Dream 1 analysis

I dreamt of a man who had his own clinic. He was in the garden, looked terrible - very big (all the proportions were not right). He had a terrible disease: the upper body was huge, the lower part of the body was like a cone, with a sinister surface. I cannot describe this at all. Do you know black spiders that carry their children on their backs? This is what this looked like. <u>Spider threads were all around him</u>. I wanted to help the man, but I didn't know how. I also couldn't diagnose what was wrong with him.

Overall, the content of the dream is evocative of a nightmare. Problem solving is present, but patient does not know how to help. The affective spectrum seems restricted to anxiety. Finally, the character in the dream displays animal-kind features indicative of poorly mature object relation.

Dream 2 analysis

It was a scary dream - I woke up full of disgust.... My mother had a baby. I was both the doctor and the father of the child. The child was strangely greenish-yellow. It did not look healthy, may have bled from the mouth. My mother did not want to know about the baby, did not want to breastfeed it. Then I gave it to her to breastfeed. Then the baby got better...

Overall, the content of the dream is still evocative of a nightmare. The patient reports his experience as scary; the dream is interrupted he wakes up full of disgust. Problem solving is present, patient now finds a solution to rescue the baby, breastfeeding helps him. The affective spectrum still seems mostly restricted to anxiety with disgust alongside. It is unsure that when the patient reported he was both doctor and father was not an observation of himself. It may possibly indicate a dissociation as in trauma. Finally, the object relation remains basic.

Dream 3 analysis

I was with my mother in a kind of barn. She wants to come to my analysis with me to listen. I promised her this at first, but then say this won't work. She says I am raping (or mutilating?) my memories. I get so angry that I grab her by the shoulders. She is light as a feather. I throw her against a table. I take off, not looking back to see if she hurt herself. I decide to go to your place (to his psychoanalysis, MLB).

By reading this excerpt, the nightmare quality is not as certain as in the first two dreams. The patient is with his mother, an object wishing to accompany him to the analysis. A proposition perceived with ambivalent feelings, is possibly indicating a maturing process of the object relation. He first agrees then retracts and the atmosphere turns gloomy and violent. Words reported are about rape, mutilation, throwing and hurting. Object relations are somewhat more mature with positive and negative appreciation of the mother, however, mostly negative. Problem solving is possibly present with the patient deciding to go and see his analyst. Anxiety is no longer in the forefront, giving way to anger. The patient is active in the dream.

Dream 4 analysis

I had a dream. I was on the phone with a woman from CH. She was the head of the Psychological Institute. During the talk she told me that a man had collapsed next to her. She told me the symptoms. Thanks to my knowledge from one of my courses at the University I diagnosed a heart attack. Since the woman did not respond, I called the emergency services myself. The person at the phone thought I was belittling him. Then I got so angry that I took care of the man myself over the phone....

With this fourth dream, we can follow the patient and call it a dream and no longer a nightmare. The patient is with an object important to him. The affective atmosphere is enlarged, with a sense of a positive relationship with the object, collaboration in saving the man who collapsed. We can also note the presence of anger. Problem solving is predominant and successful in this excerpt with the patient relying on his professional qualifications, diagnosing, calling the emergency service and finally taking care of the man himself. The patient is an actor in the dream.

## Results

From the brief analysis of the case example (Table 3.1), results using the five categories indicated a positive evolution in dreams over psychoanalysis. Results suggested less nightmares, an enlarged spectrum of affects, more successful problem-solving, with more mature object relations. Two independent raters coded the dreams with a preliminary version of the DREAMS-C, two minor discrepancies were successfully sorted after an inter-rater agreement session.[2]

From the brief example, the process of analysing the dream from an extra-clinical perspective started by taking up the words of the clinician reporting the dreams following with the examination of how they could be classified into previously defined categories. It is worth emphasizing that a few steps were needed to "translate" clinical observations into possible objects of research and saying that each step implied a simplification of the information gathered in the clinical encounter and a more abstract way of communicating the research findings. These steps are critical and may prove treacherous and call for a close collaboration between the clinician and the researcher.

*Table 3.1* Mr. X's Dream Analysis with a Preliminary Version of the DREAMS-C

| I | Nightmares | 1 | 2 | 3 | 4 |
|---|---|---|---|---|---|
| I a. | The dreamer characterizes their dream as a nightmare | ☐ | ☒ | ☐ | ☐ |
| I b. | The rater has the impression that the dreamer due to intensive fear cannot continue the dream | ☒ | ☐ | ☐ | ☐ |
| I c. | Not assessable | ☐ | ☐ | ☐ | ☐ |
| **II** | **Problem Solving** | | | | |
| II a. | Problem solution is successful | ☐ | ☒ | ☒ | ☒ |
| II b. | Problem solution is fully recognizable | ☐ | ☐ | ☐ | ☐ |
| II c. | Problem solution is partially recognizable | ☐ | ☐ | ☐ | ☐ |
| II d. | Problem solution is not recognizable | ☒ | ☐ | ☐ | ☐ |
| II e. | Not assessable | ☐ | ☐ | ☐ | ☐ |
| **III** | **Affective Spectrum** | | | | |
| III a. | Anger is present in the dream | ☐ | ☐ | ☒ | ☒ |
| III b. | Joy is present in the dream | ☐ | ☐ | ☐ | ☐ |
| III c. | Grief is present in the dream | ☐ | ☐ | ☐ | ☐ |
| III d. | Disgust is present in the dream | ☐ | ☒ | ☐ | ☐ |
| III e. | Contempt is present in the dream | ☐ | ☐ | ☐ | ☐ |
| III f. | Fear is present in the dream | ☐ | ☒ | ☐ | ☐ |
| III g. | Surprise is present in the dream | ☐ | ☐ | ☐ | ☐ |
| III h. | Other affects are present in the dream. Specify: _____ | ☐ | ☐ | ☐ | ☐ |
| III i. | No affects are present in the dream | ☒ | ☐ | ☐ | ☐ |
| III j. | Not assessable | ☐ | ☐ | ☐ | ☐ |
| **IV** | **Self-Agency** | | | | |
| IV a. | The patient is an actor in the dream | ☐ | ☒ | ☒ | ☒ |
| IV b. | The patient is an "outside" observer of the dream action | ☐ | ☐ | ☐ | ☐ |
| IV c. | The patient is present in the dream, but passive | ☒ | ☐ | ☐ | ☐ |
| IV d. | The patient is present in the dream, but paralyzed | ☐ | ☐ | ☐ | ☐ |
| IV e. | Not assessable | ☐ | ☐ | ☐ | ☐ |

## Conclusion

Starting from findings of the LAC study, the MODE study was theoretically grounded in a perspective of special benefits of intensive psychoanalytic treatment for patients with chronic depression and early trauma. The detailed clinical observations of the clinician-researchers participating to the LAC study put them in a position to make suggestions for refining the theoretical context for the treatment of chronic depression in patients with early trauma (Leuzinger-Bohleber et al., 2022). In the MODE study, the detailed case study allows for further theory building, Leuzinger-Bohleber's detailed clinical observations brought her in a position to make suggestions to refine the theoretical background as well as support changes in dreams as a means to report on the process of change in an intensive psychoanalysis with a young adult with an arrested development. When examined from a research perspective, the dream material revealed a positive evolution over the psychoanalysis. Thanks to the clinician-researcher collaboration, the instrument used here may offer a possibility to systematically investigate clinical suggestions in the dream diaries collected in the MODE study, hopefully from 100 psychoanalyses. The examination of the "accumulated observations" collected through detailed case studies will allow them to contribute to the refinement of the theory guiding the treatment of patients with chronic depression and early trauma. Hence, the MODE study will offer an opportunity to make the worlds of words and of stats meet. Clinicians and researchers will then be in a position to gain knowledge greater than the two parts.

## Notes

1  In this scale, we are integrating the Dreams-Content Analyses of Leuzinger-Bohleber (1989), the ZDPCS (by Moser & von Zeppelin, 1996) and the SCROS-G (Stein & Slavin-Mulford, 2017). In several pilot studies (master theses by Nicolette Zuccarini, Paula Rehm and Lea Scholz) the reliability of the Scale has been investigated. Reliability and validity tests are still ongoing (Leuzinger-Bohleber et al., in print).
2  We are especially thankful to Nicoletta Zuccarini for her participation in coding the dreams.

## Bibliography

Altmann de Litvan, M. (ed.) (2014) *Time for change*. London: Karnac.

Blos, P. (1967). The second individuation process in adolescence. *Psychoanalytic Study of the Child, 22*, 162–187.

Bohleber, W. (2010). *Destructiveness, intersubjectivity and trauma: The identity crisis of modern psychoanalysis*. London: Karnac Books.

Bohleber, W., & Leuzinger-Bohleber, M. (1981). Narzissmus und Adoleszenz. In Psychoanalytisches Seminar Zürich (Hg.) *Die neuen Narzissmustheorien. Zurück ins Paradies?* Frankfurt a.M.: Syndikat, p. 117.

Campbell, D.T. (1979). "Degrees of freedom" and the case study. In Cook, T.D., & Reichardt, C.S. (eds.) *Qualitative and quantitative methods in evaluation research* (Vol. 1). Beverly Hills, CA: Sage publications, pp. 49–67.

Chasseguet-Smirgel, J. (1991). Sadomasochism in the perversions: Some thoughts on the destruction of reality. *Journal of the American Psychoanalytic Association, 39*(2), 399–415.

Fischmann, T., Ambresin, G., & Leuzinger-Bohleber, M. (2021). Dreams and trauma changes in the manifest dreams in psychoanalytic treatments–A psychoanalytic outcome measure. *Frontiers in Psychology, 12*, 678440

Fishman, D.B., Messer, S.B., Edwards, D.J., & Dattilio, F.M. (eds.) (2016). *Case studies within psychotherapy trials: Integrating qualitative and quantitative methods*. New York: Oxford University Press.

Fitzpatrick Hanly, M.A., Altmann de Litvan, M., & Bernardi, R. (eds.) (2021). *Change through time in psychoanalysis transformations and interventions, the three level model*. London: Routledge.

Freud, A. (1958). Adolescence. In Freud, A. (ed.). *The writings of Anna Freud* (Vol. 5). New York: International Universities Press, pp. 136–166.

Freud, A. (1965). *Normality and psychopathology in childhood*. New York: International University Press.

Freud, S. (1900). In Strachey, J. (ed.) *The standard edition of the complete psychological works of Sigmund Freud* (Vol. 4/5), pp. 1–627. London: Hogarth Press.

Freud, S. (1933). New introductory lectures on psycho-analysis. In Strachey, J. (ed.) *The standard edition of the complete psychological works of Sigmund Freud* (Vol. 22), pp. 1–182. London: Hogarth Press.

Freud, S. (1937). Analysis terminable and interminable. In Strachey, J. (ed.) *The standard edition of the complete psychological works of Sigmund Freud* (Vol. 23), pp 216–257. London: Hogarth Press.

Green, A. (2003). The pluralism of sciences and psychoanalytic thinking. In Leuzinger-Bohleber, M.E., Dreher, A.U., Canestri, J. (eds.) *Pluralism and unity?* London: Routledge, pp. 26–44.

Gullestad, S.E., & Killingmo, B. (2020). *The theory and practice of psychoanalytic therapy: Listening for the subtext*. London:Routledge.

Kächele, H. (2020). From case study to single case research: The specimen case Amalia X. In Leuzinger-Bohleber, M.E., Solms, M.E., & Arnold, S.E. (eds.) *Outcome research and the future of psychoanalysis*. Routledge/Taylor & Francis Group. Psychoanalysis, pp. 68–88.

Kächele, H., Albani, C., Pokorny, D. (2015). From a psychoanalytic narrative case study to quantitative single-case research. In Gelo, O.C.G., Pritz, A., & Riegen, B. (eds.) *Psychotherapy research – Foundations, process and outcome*. Wien: Springer-Verlag, pp. 367–379.

Kaechele, H. (2012): Dreams as subject of psychoanalytic treatement research.In Fonagy, P., Kaechele, H., Leuzinger-Bohleber, M., Taylor, D. (eds): The Significance of Dreams. London: Routledge, 89–101.

Lemma, A. (2010). An order of pure decision: Growing up in a virtual world and the adolescent's experience of being-in-a-body. *Journal of the American Psychoanalytic Association*, *58*(4), 691–714.

Leuzinger-Bohleber, M. (2015). Working with severely traumatized, chronically depressed analysands. *The International Journal of Psychoanalysis*, *96*(3), 611–636.

Leuzinger-Bohleber, M. (1987). Veränderung kognitiver Prozesse in Psychoanalysen. In Leuzinger-Bohleber, M. (ed.) *Bd. 1: Eine hypothesengenerierende Einzelfallstudie*. Berlin: Springer (PSZ), pp. 1–428.

Leuzinger-Bohleber, M. (1989). Veränderung kognitiver Prozesse in Psychoanalysen. In Leuzinger-Bohleber, M. (ed.) *Bd. 2: Fünf aggregierte Einzelfallstudien*. Berlin: Springer (PSZ), pp. 1–536.

Leuzinger-Bohleber, M. (2000). Wandering between the worlds – From an analysis of a late adolescent. In Klitzing, K.v., Tyson, P., & Bürgin, D. (eds.) *Psychoanalysis in childhood and adolescence*. New York: Karger, pp. 104–125.

Leuzinger-Bohleber, M. (2018). Finding the body in the mind: Embodiment and approaching the non-represented—A case study and some theory. In Leuzinger-Bohleber, M. (Ed.) *Finding the body in the mind*. London: Routledge, pp. 19–31.

Leuzinger-Bohleber, M. (2020). Una investigación de los cambios sintomáticos y estructurales en el studio LAC de la depresión. Hallazgos empíricos y clínicos. *Revista de Psicoanálisis*, *77*(12), 223–249.

Leuzinger-Bohleber, M. (2023). "Il fili di ragno lo circondavano.." Lánalisi´ad alte frequenza´ è una buona scelta per gli arresti evolutivi nello "stato adulto emergente"?. *Rivista di Psicoanalisi, LXIX*(2), 1–26.

Leuzinger-Bohleber, M., Ambresin, G., Fischmann, T., & Solms, M. (eds.) (2022). *On the dark side of chronic depression: Psychoanalytic, social-cultural and research approaches*. London: Taylor & Francis.

Leuzinger-Bohleber, M., & Arnold, S.E. (2020). Introduction: Outcome research and the future of psychoanalysis. In Leuzinger-Bohleber, M., Solms, M., & Arnold, S.E. (eds.) *Outcome research and the future of psychoanalysis. Clinicans and researchers in dialogue.* London: Routledge, pp. 1–26.

Leuzinger-Bohleber, M., Fischmann, T., & Beutel, M.E. (2022). *Chronische depression: Analytische langzeitpsychotherapie* (Vol. 12). Bern: Hogrefe Verlag GmbH & Company KG.

Leuzinger-Bohleber, M., Grabhorn, A., & Bahrke, U. (2020). *Was nur erzählt und nicht gemessen werden kann. Einblicke in psychoanalytische Langzeitbehandlungen chronischer Depressionen.* Gießen: Psychosozial-Verlag.

Leuzinger-Bohleber, M., Hautzinger, M., Fiedler, G., Keller, W., Bahrke, U., Kallenbach, L., … & Küchenhoff, H. (2019a). Outcome of psychoanalytic and cognitive-behavioural long-term therapy with chronically depressed patients: A controlled trial with preferential and randomized allocation. *The Canadian Journal of Psychiatry, 64*(1), pp. 47–58.

Leuzinger-Bohleber, M., & Kächele, H. (eds.) (2015). *An open door review of outcome and process studies in psychoanalysis.* London: International Psychoanalytical Association.

Leuzinger-Bohleber, M., Kallenbach, L., Bahrke, U., Kaufhold, J., Negele, A., Ernst, M., & Beutel, M.E. (2020). The LAC Study: A comparative outcome study of psychoanalytic and cognitive-behavioral long-term therapies of chronic depressive patients. In Leuzinger-Bohleber, M.E., Solms, M.E., & Arnold, S.E. (eds.) *Outcome research and the future of psychoanalysis.* Outcome research and the future of psychoanalysis: Clinicians and researchers in dialogue. Routledge/Taylor & Francis Group, pp. 136–165.

Leuzinger-Bohleber, M., Kallenbach, L., & Schoett, M.J.S. (2016). Pluralistic approaches to the study of process and outcome in psychoanalysis. The LAC depression study: A case in point. *Psychoanalytic Psychotherapy, 30*(1), 4–22. DOI: 10.1080/02668734.2015.1107123.

Leuzinger-Bohleber, M., Kaufhold, J., Kallenbach, L., Negele, A., Ernst, M., Keller, W., … & Beutel, M. (2019b). How to measure sustained psychic transformations in long-term treatments of chronically depressed patients: Symptomatic and structural changes in the LAC Depression Study of the outcome of cognitive-behavioural and psychoanalytic long-term treatments. *The International Journal of Psychoanalysis, 100*(1), 99–127.

Leuzinger-Bohleber, M., & Westenberger-Breuer, H. (2020, September). Was nur erzählt und nicht gemessen werden kann. In Leuzinger-Bohleber, M., Grabhorn, A., Bahrke, U. (eds) *Was nur erzählt und nicht gemessen werden kann.* Psychosozial-Verlag, pp. 9–82.

Leuzinger-Bohleber, M., Donié M, Wichelmann, J., Ambresin, G., Fischmann, T. (accepted). Changes in dreams - the development of a dream-transformation scale in psychoanalyses with chronically depressed, early traumatized patients. *Scandinavian Psychoanalytic Review*

Luyten, P. (2012). Commentary: The coming of age of psychoanalytic treatment research. In *Psychodynamic psychotherapy research*. Totowa, NJ: Humana Press, pp. 337–343.

Makari, G. (2008). *Revolution in mind: The creation of psychoanalysis*. London: Duckworth & Co.

Moser, U., & von Zeppelin, I. (1996). *Der geträumte Traum. Wie Träume entstehen und sich verändern*. Stuttgart: Kohlhammer.

Seiffge-Krenke, I. & Weitkamp, K. (2020). How individual coping, mental health, and parental behavior is related to identity development in emerging adults in seven countries. *Emerging Adulthood, 8*(5), 344–360.

Stein, M., & Slavin-Mulford, J. (2017). *The social cognition and object relations scale-global rating method (SCORS-G): A comprehensive guide for clinicians and researchers*. London: Routledge.

Stiles, W.B. (2009). Logical operations in theory-building case studies. *Pragmatic Case Studies in Psychotherapy, 5*(3), 9–22.

Thurin, J.M. (2017). From the evaluation of psychotherapies to research in psychotherapy and psychoanalysis. *Research in Psychoanalysis*, (1), 55–68.

Wallerstein, R. (1986). *Forty-two lives in treatment. A study of psychoanalysis and psychotherapy*. New York: The Analytic Press.

Winnicott, D.W. (1971). *Playing and reality*. New York: Basic Books, Inc.

# 4 In Kandel's footsteps

## Epigenetics and therapeutic change

*Juan Pablo Jiménez and Yamil Quevedo*

### Introducing Midap or how to build a psychoanalytically relevant research center from scratch… in 30 years

Our research group started 30 years ago at a first research meeting that brought together a small group of psychoanalysts and young psychologists from Chile, Argentina, and Uruguay interested in psychotherapy research. This meeting, which had the support and attendance of Horst Kächele (Ulm, Germany) and Kenn Howard (Chicago, USA), was the origin of the Latin American Chapter of the *Society for Psychotherapy Research*. In 30 years, the group grew in number and quality. To improve the quality of our research, in 2007 we founded the PhD program in Psychotherapy, a joint program between the University of Chile, the Pontifical Catholic University of Chile, and the University of Heidelberg in Germany. To foster dialogue with clinicians, we founded the Chilean Congress of Psychotherapy, which brings together researchers and clinicians. In the years that followed, our group earned various funding for research projects. Finally, in 2014 we managed to win the *Millennium Institute for Research in Depression and Personality*, Midap, from the Millennium Science Initiative Programme, which only funds scientific proposals of international excellence. Midap has been highly productive, in terms of publications in high-impact journals, in training advanced human capital, and in disseminating its findings to society, which are the basis for future public policies.

We believe that the key to our success has been the research strategy. Unlike psychotherapy research centers in the Global North, and even though most of our researchers were and still are clinically trained therapists in the psychodynamic orientation, our strategy focused not on advocating the superiority of one psychotherapeutic orientation but on exploring the factors common to all forms of psychotherapy. In this way, we encouraged collaboration rather than competition between orientations. One of our central aims has been to develop a model of psychotherapy that could be applied in the public health system, beyond the private practice of therapists, that is empirically sound (Jiménez & de la Parra, 2023).

DOI: 10.4324/9781032651934-6

## The impact of early trauma on adult psychopathology

### Freud's break with the etiopathogenic theory of degeneration, the prevailing theory 100 years ago

Freud's arrival in France in 1885 brought him face to face with the theory of degeneration, formulated by Auguste Morel in 1850. After this theory the "degenerate" had a family history that justified his illness – epilepsy, alcoholism, sexually transmitted diseases, prostitution, neuropathies, and insanity – and his body had well-defined features, the stigmata, which were perfectly recognizable to the doctor's eye.

However, we know of Freud's opposition to such a theory of degeneration. Taking advantage of scientific field tilting against Charcot, Freud also threw himself against degeneration theory. Freud thought that the theory of *famille névropathique* was in desperate need of reevaluation. In footnotes of his translation of Charcot's articles, Freud made it clear that he considered Charcot wrong about the hereditary nature of hysteria. In fact, he confessed that he considered hysteria to be solely the result of trauma (Makari, 2008).

The vicissitudes of the concept of trauma in the more than 100 years of history of psychoanalysis are well known, its initial boom and its passing into the background, sometimes almost disappearing, only to reappear again in contemporary theories. In any case, the central idea of the mode of action of psychoanalytic treatment of traumatized patients is that trauma awareness enables individuals to integrate repressed traumatic memories into mental life and thus form new ways of coping with them. However, it took 100 years before the pathophysiological mechanism of early trauma and the psychobiological mechanisms of action of psychotherapy could be scientifically studied.

### What do we mean by early trauma?

The concept of early life stress is broad and includes stressful and/or traumatic experiences occurring during childhood and adolescence, such as family violence, separation from parents, lack of food, shelter, love, etc. Studies on the effects of child abuse include acts of physical, sexual, and emotional abuse and episodes of physical and emotional neglect. Broadly speaking, abuse – whether physical, sexual, or psychological – is a form of intentional abuse, while neglect – emotional or physical – corresponds to parents' failure to meet children's basic needs. There are several psychometric instruments that are used to assess perceptions of early life adversity; we used the Child Trauma Questionnaire-Short Form (CTQ-SF).

### What do we know about the impact of early trauma on adult psychopathology?

There is an abundant scientific literature on the effect of early life stress in adult physical and mental illness. The shocking title of "The Devastating

Clinical Consequences of Child Abuse and Neglect…" (Lippard & Ne-meroff, 2020) speaks for itself. In relation to the global impact of early life stress in adulthood, there are some general facts: It is already known that exposure to one or more *Adverse Childhood Experiences* (ACEs) related to abuse accounts for 54% of the population's attributable risk of depression, 67% of the attributable risk of suicide attempts, and 64% of the attributable risk of illicit drug addiction. Exposure to five or more adverse experiences was associated with an increase of 2, 3, 10, or 17 times in the risk of receiving a prescription of an anxiolytic, antidepressant, antipsychotic, or mood-stabilizing medication, respectively. Individuals exposed to six or more ACEs have a reduction of 20 years in useful life (Teicher et al., 2016). We can conclude that understanding how maltreatment increases the risk of various psychiatric (and medical) disorders is of crucial importance in preventing and treating the consequences of early abuse and neglect.

### Our findings in a non-clinical sample

What do our own findings tell us in this respect? In a non-clinical sample of 673 young university students from Santiago and Temuco, we found that 44.7% of participants reported early trauma on at least one CTQ subscale. Disaggregated by each, 27.8% suffered emotional abuse, 16.8% physical abuse, and 12% sexual abuse. On the other hand, 10.1% reported physical neglect while 7.1% reported emotional neglect during childhood.

In the same sample, 28.1% of the recruited students reported depressive symptoms measured by the Beck self-report scale (BDI-I). These results agree with national and international research findings, which show higher rates in university students compared to the general population, with coincidences in the report regarding the greater presence of depressive symptoms in women.

In order to know the association between depressive symptomatology and early stress in our students, we evaluated the existence of significant associations between the average score obtained in the Beck Depression Inventory (BDI) and the level of early trauma obtained in each of the subscales of the CTQ. On all CTQ scales, we found significant associations with important levels of depressive symptomatology, beyond the cut-off point of established clinical significance (Rossi et al., 2019).

### Childhood maltreatment and its role in the clinical course of patients with bipolar disorder

This was a non-clinical population sample. But we also have data from a clinical population. We studied 101 type I bipolar euthymic patients, i.e., without acute states of depression or mania. Of the 101 patients, 64% had some form of child abuse or neglect, 42% were victims of sexual abuse, 30% were victims of physical abuse, 23% were victims of emotional abuse.

10% were victims of three types of abuse (physical, sexual, and emotional), 17% were victims of two types of abuse, 31% were victims of one type of abuse (Ríos et al., 2020). From the international literature, we know that as adults, patients who have a mental illness such as depression or bipolar disorder and who have suffered trauma in vulnerable periods tend to have an earlier onset, more difficult course, and worse response to treatment. Most intriguing, in bipolar patients, psychological trauma makes them more refractory to treatment with lithium, a biological therapy. Our findings are comparable with international studies showing that patients with bipolar disorder report high levels of childhood maltreatment (Hyun et al., 2000; Romero et al., 2009), with estimates as high as 57% (Post et al., 2013). We must think that, as a result of trauma, plasticity or prosocial genes are modified in their expression by epigenetic mechanisms.

The findings of the German study conducted by Marianne Leuzinger-Bohleber in chronic depressive treatment refractory patients, show even more dramatic results. 75.7% reported having suffered some type of significant trauma (Leuzinger-Bohleber, 2015).

With these data, we can claim that the more severe the trauma, the more severe the depression in adulthood and the more difficult its treatment.

## Epigenetics: the action of the (human) environment on gene expression

### Epigenetics as a mechanism of gene-environment interaction

With his study on the effect of learning on synaptic changes in the marine snail of the genus Aplysia, Eric Kandel won the Nobel Prize in Medicine and Physiology in 2000. With his research he opened the way to understanding how psychotherapy produces molecular changes, at the level of gene expression. However, the road from snail research to human beings is a long and difficult one.

Psychotherapy is a process that brings about changes in an individual's behavior, thereby modifying his or her experiences and interaction with the environment. As Eric Kandel (1998, 1999, 2001) has argued, effective psychotherapy also produces alterations in gene expression which, in turn, produce structural changes in the brain. Kandel stresses the importance of procedural memory in the context of emotion and understanding of what happens in the transference relationship during the therapeutic process. Psychotherapy modifies synapses. These changes that occur within the transference relationship do not necessarily require the unconscious to become conscious, but rather the acquisition of a new set of implicit memories that in turn lead to behavioral changes that increase the range of procedural strategies for further progress, in the sense of new strategies for action that are reflected in the way the person interacts with others. Kandel's research has given a biological meaning to the Freudian concept of *psychotherapy as after-education* (*Nacherziehung*). With our research on human beings, we follow in Kandel's footsteps.

In this way, activation of epigenetic processes allows that social and environmental experiences, both positive and negative, are transformed into persistent changes in behavior, in other words, the phenotypic adaptation to a changing environment (Slavich & Cole, 2013).

Epigenetic mechanisms are stable changes of potential gene expression during development and cell proliferation that are held through cell divisions and do not alter the DNA sequence (Jaenisch & Bird, 2003). There are several specific mechanisms such as heritable patterns of DNA methylation and hydroxymethylation, post-translational histone modifications, and non-coding RNAs (Zannas, 2016).

The unique way in which genes are expressed is influenced by various processes, and this pattern is not fixed, but rather subject to change in response to environmental factors. It is also diverse among different organisms, tissues, and cells and can vary throughout different stages of development and life cycles. This mechanism of "phenotypic plasticity" enables organisms to adapt to environmental demands (Weaver, 2007).

There are three forms of relationship between the environment and epigenetic changes, which are not mutually exclusive: (a) a socio-environmental explanation that, environmental stimuli are maintained for a long time; (b) a socio-cognitive explanation in which the stressor can last a short time, but its effect is mediated by the continuity of cognitive processing it, for example, experiences of loneliness and isolation after breakup of a relationship persists; and (c) a biological explanation indicates that exposure occurs at critical developmental windows and allow the "remodeling of the transcriptional dynamics" (Slavich & Cole, 2013). The latter mechanism is also known as "biological embedding" in which the neurobiological adaptations vary according to the intensity and quality of early experiences (Lutz & Turecki, 2014).

In humans, adverse early experiences can also exert their influence on behavioral patterns and psychiatric disorders in adulthood through epigenetic modifications. In subjects who reported various adverse events during her childhood, including physical, emotional, and sexual abuse, a correlation is found between the number of adverse events reported and methylation of a specific site of the glucocorticoid receptor gene. Additionally, this pattern is correlated with the presence of borderline symptoms (Radtke et al., 2011).

In a sample of adopted individuals, the Berkeley Attachment Interview (AAI), a semi-structured interview, was administered to assess the presence of unresolved trauma or loss. Higher levels of DNA methylation in the promoter region of the serotonin transporter gene 5HTT were associated with an increased risk of unresolved trauma in carriers of a specific phenotype I/I ("long alleles", usually considered "protector"). These interactions suggest a mediation between the adverse emotional environment and methylation in phenotypic development (van IJzendoorn et al., 2010).

*Can subjective processes affect molecular mechanisms?*

Kendler (2005) states that subjective or "first-person" experiences have causal efficacy in the organism and are highly elaborate forms of intentional processes that eventually lead to action. Mental disorders are related to the failure of these intentional states to exert adaptation. Fonagy et al. (2004) argue that the intrapsychic representational processes can moderate the effects of the environment on the phenotype; in other words, the interpretation of the social environment acts on the genetic expression as a mechanism of adaptation of the phenotype.

The subjective perception of the social environment (e.g., perception of isolation or social anxiety) can act at different biological systems, such as the central nervous system, hypothalamic pituitary adrenal axis, intracellular signaling, and genetic expression. Slavich and Cole (2013) call this process "social signal transduction". A study exemplifying this was conducted by assessing self-reported perception of social rejection in adolescents. An increase in inflammatory markers was associated with greater perceived social rejection. One possible explanation is that when faced with a threat to their social status, molecular mechanisms are activated that prepare the individual to face a potential physical aggression (Murphy et al., 2013).

Mentalization can be understood as the mental activity that allows us to interpret human social behavior in terms of intentional mental states (needs, desires, feelings, goals), constituting a form of social cognition (Fonagy & Luyten, 2009). This capability is an achievement of development, a result of an evolutionary process, which in turn depends on early experiences and the emotional bond that is formed with a caregiver. It is crucial for the development of mentalization, the quality of early attachment relationships, as they allow the internal states to be mirrored by an attentive and reliable caretaker, this process at the same time impacts the processes of emotional regulation and self-control (Fonagy & Luyten, 2009).

The "Social Brain Network" (dorsal medial prefrontal cortex, temporoparietal junction, posterior superior temporal sulcus, and anterior temporal cortex) underlies various forms of socioemotional processing such as mentalizing, social emotion, and peer evaluation and remains in development until early adulthood (Blakemore, 2013). This makes adolescence a "sensitive period" open to social interactions that act as a critical input for human social development.

Jablonka and Lamb (2006) have described the mechanism of "social mediated learning", which is the acquisition of knowledge from the social milieu to ensure survival and mating. In humans, the symbolic transmission of information through language configures a new system of non-genetic inheritance, in addition to genetic, epigenetic, and behavioral dimensions of inheritance that interact with each other in the configuration of the phenotype.

Epigenetic mechanisms are both permeable to environmental influences and stable over time so it is possible to argue that they can be a mechanism for long-term effects on the social brain network and its social cognition functions such as mentalization, of both early experiences and significant emotional experiences, such as psychotherapy, in sensitive periods of life.

## Epigenetics and psychotherapy

Only a few studies address the potential link between epigenetic changes and diverse types of psychotherapy: for example, in exposure therapy for post-traumatic stress disorder and cognitive behavioral therapy for panic disorders. A limited number of studies have explored the effect of psychotherapy on epigenetic changes in borderline personality disorder (BPD).

One study using a sample of outpatients diagnosed with BPD measured DNA methylation of *BDNF* gene before and after four weeks of intensive dialectical behavioral psychotherapy (DBT). Patients, who responded to DBT, exhibited a decrease in DNA methylation of *BDNF* gene (Perroud et al., 2013). In another study, individuals with BPD who responded to DBT therapy presented higher DNA methylation in *APBA3* and *MCF2* genes after 12 weeks relative to non-responders (Knoblich et al., 2017). A third study reported a decrease in DNA methylation levels of *BDNF* after 12 weeks of DBT (Thomas et al., 2018). These initial findings suggest that psychotherapy may influence peripheral DNA methylation levels and could be considered as a potential biomarker of psychotherapy improvement.

To explore the relationship between epigenetic changes and psychotherapy in adolescents with BPD, our group conducted a longitudinal pilot study (Quevedo et al., 2022). Specifically, we measure changes in DNA methylation of *FKBP5* gene, which encodes for a stress response protein, in relation to psychotherapy in a sample of 11 female adolescents diagnosed with BPD.

A significant reduction of borderline and depressive symptoms was found. A reduction in the average FKBP5 DNA methylation was observed over time. Additionally, it was observed that this decrease in methylation occurred only in those individuals who reported the presence of early trauma and responded to psychotherapy.

These results highlight the potential role of psychotherapy as capable of exerting actions at the epigenetic level on genes associated with stress response in individuals with BPD, specifically DNA methylation of FKBP5, which is concordant with the results of previous studies in PTSD, children with anxiety disorders and individuals with Agoraphobia. Bishop et al. (2018) also report significant findings in individuals with PTSD treated with Mindfulness Based Stress Reduction therapy, but in the opposite direction. DBT psychotherapy has previously been associated with DNA methylation change in other genes in BPD subjects, but not with *FKBP5* (Perroud et al., 2013; Knoblich et al., 2017; Thomas et al., 2018).

### Concluding remarks: limitations of our study and future research

In our pilot study, only individuals who reported the presence of early trauma and who responded to psychotherapy exhibited a decrease in DNA methylation. This differential response by the presence of early trauma is suggestive of a specific mechanism of recovery. In this sample, the differential response to psychotherapy at the level of DNA methylation may imply that some individuals are more permeable at the molecular level to both negative (early trauma) and positive influences (psychotherapy) from their affective environment.

According to the differential sensitivity model, individuals carrying "plasticity genes" faced with an early suboptimal affective environment, would be more susceptible to develop psychopathology but can be also more susceptible to respond to positive social environments (Hammen et al., 2000).

In accordance with the above, a Genome-wide association study (GWAS) of twins reported a polygenic score based on differences in sensitivity to develop anxiety disorders according to positive or negative parenting. In a second sample, individuals with a major differential sensitivity polygenic score responded better to individual cognitive behavioral therapy (Keers et al., 2016). These results suggest that those individuals who present a greater sensitivity to the environment present more emotional problems if they experienced negative parenting, but they will also be the ones who will benefit most from psychotherapy.

The formation of an alliance between patient and therapist can lead to the restoration of "epistemic trust", which restores an individual's confidence in obtaining knowledge relevant to their adaptation to the social world from another human being (Fonagy & Allison, 2014). This is particularly relevant for individuals with BPD, as insecure attachment patterns developed in suboptimal interaction with their caregivers involve chronic epistemic mistrust with the concomitant development of deficient behavioral and emotional patterns for establishing cooperation and the ability to repair ruptures in relationships with others.

Psychotherapy is a biologically embedded experience capable of altering biological functions in a stable and long-term manner. In animal models, social plasticity is achieved by structural reorganization or biochemical switching of relevant neural circuits of neural networks underlying social behavior in response to perceived social information (Cardoso et al., 2015). Psychotherapy can modify the configuration of neural systems of emotional regulation, social cognition, and impulsivity, changing both brain activity and structure. Reprogramming gene expression of molecules attached to key biological systems of neurotransmission, neuromodulation, neuroplasticity, and stress response (Jiménez et al., 2018). Psychotherapy can be understood as a disrupter of the "external social recursion" that goes from the social environment to neural systems, modifying the subjective perception of the interpersonal environment, and capable of informing and changing the "internal physiologic recursion" that ranges from the Central Nervous System to gene expression, including hormonal systems, inflammatory molecules, and intracellular signal transduction (Slavich & Cole, 2013).

In individuals with BPD, an effective patient-therapist relationship can lead to stable changes in the mentalizing neural network and a reduction in rigid and maladaptive responses of hyperactivation or deactivation of attachment patterns, resulting in greater reflective awareness of one's own state of mind (Luyten & Fonagy, 2015; Herpertz et al., 2018). DNA methylation, a stable epigenetic marker, can be used to assess changes in personality functioning over time, especially during critical windows of development, such as adolescence. Psychotherapy can positively affect the processing of interpersonal information through new meaningful relational experiences, leading to improvements in the ability to reflect on emotional states and interpersonal experiences and regulation of affects, behavior, and relationships.

To conduct effective epigenetic studies in psychopathology, researchers should use a refined and replicable characterization of both the phenotype to be studied and the psychotherapeutic intervention. Researchers can also use intermediate phenotypes or endophenotypes, such as social cognition, neuroimaging, hormonal, and inflammatory markers, to explore the interrelationship between multiple explanatory levels. Other process measures can be incorporated, such as the therapeutic alliance (Horvath et al., 2011).

Our results should be taken with caution given the small sample size. Further research requires longitudinal, prospective study designs, with adequate statistical power and the use of repeated measures to explore the interaction between different aspects of the psychotherapy and DNA methylation changes throughout the therapy process. Ideally, researchers should obtain data from multiple tissues to quantify cross-tissue correlation, and in the future, capture the methylome broadly, including not only methylation but also non-coding RNAs and histone modifications (Barker et al., 2017).

## References

Barker, E. D., Walton, E., Cecil, C. A. M., & Viding, E. (2017). Epigenetics and child psychopathology: current insights and future directions. *Journal of Child Psychology and Psychiatry*, 58(4), 387–392.

Bishop, J. R., Lee, A. M., Mills, L. J., Thuras, P. D., Eum, S., Clancy, D., et al. (2018). Methylation of FKBP5 and SLC6A4 in relation to treatment response to mindfulness-based stress reduction for posttraumatic stress disorder. *Frontiers in Psychiatry*, 9, 418. doi: 10.3389/fpsyt.2018.00418.

Blakemore, S. J. (2013). Imaging brain development: the adolescent brain. *Neuroimage*, 61(2), 397–406.

Cardoso, S. D., Teles, M. C., & Oliveira, R. F. (2015). Neurogenomic mechanisms of social plasticity. *The Journal of Experimental Biology*, 218(Pt 1), 140–149. https:// doi.org/10.1242/jeb.106997.

Fonagy, P., & Allison, E. (2014). The role of mentalizing and epistemic trust in the therapeutic relationship. *Psychotherapy*, 51(3), 372–380. doi: 10.1037/a0036505.

Fonagy, P., Gergely, G., & Jurist, E. L. (2004). *Affect regulation, mentalization, and the development of the self.* Other Press.

Fonagy, P., & Luyten, P. (2009). A developmental, mentalization-based approach to the understanding and treatment of borderline personality disorder. *Development and Psychopathology*, 21(4), 1355–1381.

Hammen, C., Henry, R., & Daley, S. E. (2000). Depression and sensitization to stressors among young women as a function of childhood adversity. *Journal of Consulting and Clinical Psychology*, 68(5), 782–787. doi: 10.1037/0022-006X.68.5.782.

Herpertz, S. C., Bertsch, K., & Ogrodniczuk, J. S. (2018). The role of the psychotherapeutic relationship in the treatment of personality disorders. *American Journal of Psychiatry*, 175(5), 428-436.

Horvath, A. O., Del Re, A. C., Flückiger, C., & Symonds, D. (2011). Alliance in individual psychotherapy. *Psychotherapy*, 48, 9–16. doi: 10.1037/a0022186.

Hyun, M., Friedman, S. D., & Dunner, D. L. (2000). Relationship of childhood physical and sexual abuse to adult bipolar disorder. *Bipolar Disorder*, 2, 131–135.

Jablonka, E., & Lamb, M. J. (2006). The evolution of information in the major transitions. *Journal of Theoretical Biology*, 239(2), 236–246.

Jaenisch, R., & Bird, A. (2003). Epigenetic regulation of gene expression: how the genome integrates intrinsic and environmental signals. *Nature Genetics*, 33(3), 245–254.

Jiménez, J. P., Botto, A., Herrera, L., Leighton, C., Rossi, J. L., Quevedo, Y., et al. (2018). Psychotherapy and genetic neuroscience: an emerging dialog. *Frontiers in Genetics*, 9, 257. doi: 10.3389/fgene.2018.00257.

Jiménez, J. P., & de la Parra, G. (2023). A long but fruitful journey: From clinical psychoanalysis to public mental health in Chile. *International Journal of Applied Psychoanalytic Studies*, 20(2), 302–315. https://doi-org.pucdechile.idm.oclc. org/10.1002/aps.1815.

Kandel, E. R. (1998). A new intellectual framework for psychiatry. *The American Journal of Psychiatry*, 155, 457–469. doi: 10.1176/ajp.155.4.457.

Kandel, E. R. (1999). Biology and the future of psychoanalysis: a new intellectual framework for psychiatry revisited. *The American Journal of Psychiatry*, 156, 505–524.

Kandel, E. R. (2001). The molecular biology of memory storage: a dialog between genes and synapses. *Bioscience Reports*, 21, 565–611. doi: 10.1023/A:1014775008533.

Keers, R., Coleman, J. R., Lester, K. J., Roberts, S., Breen, G., Thastum, M., et al. (2016). A genome-wide test of the differential susceptibility hypothesis reveals a genetic predictor of differential response to psychological treatments for child anxiety disorders. *Psychotherapy and Psychosomatics*, 85(3), 146–158. doi: 10.1159/000442854.

Kendler, K. S. (2005). Toward a philosophical structure for psychiatry. *The American Journal of Psychiatry*, 162(3), 433–440.

Knoblich, S., Paul, T., Dainese, S. M., Singer, F., Stäblein, M., Schicktanz, N., et al. (2017). DNA methylation in a distressed young population: association with severity and clinical characteristics. *Journal of Psychiatric Research*, 84, 254–262. doi: 10.1016/j.jpsychires.2016.10.001.

Leuzinger-Bohleber, M. (2015). Working with severely traumatized, chronically depressed analysands. *The International Journal of Psychoanalysis*, 96, 611–636.

Lippard, E. T. C., & Nemeroff, C. B. (2020). The devastating clinical consequences of child abuse and neglect: increased disease vulnerability and poor treatment response in mood disorders. *The American Journal of Psychiatry*, 177(1), 20–36. https://doi.org/10.1176/appi.ajp.2019.19010020.

Lutz, P. E., & Turecki, G. (2014). DNA methylation and childhood maltreatment: from animal models to human studies. *Neuroscience*, 264, 142–156.

Luyten, P., & Fonagy, P. (2015). The neurobiology of mentalizing. *Personality Disorders*, 6(4), 366–379. https://doi.org/10.1037/per0000117.

Makari, G. (2008). *Revolution in Mind: The Creation of Psychoanalysis*. New York: Harper Collins Publishers.

Murphy, M. L., Slavich, G. M., Rohleder, N., & Miller, G. E. (2013). Targeted rejection triggers differential pro- and anti-inflammatory gene expression in adolescents as a function of social status. *Clinical Psychological Science: A Journal of the Association for Psychological Science*, 1(1), 30–40. https://doi.org/10.1177/2167702612455743

Perroud, N., Dayer, A., Piguet, C., Nallet, A., Favre, S., Malafosse, A., et al. (2013). Childhood maltreatment and methylation of the glucocorticoid receptor gene NR3C1 in bipolar disorder. *The British Journal of Psychiatry*, 204(1), 30–35. doi: 10.1192/bjp.bp.112.121667.

Post, R. M., Altshuler, L., Leverich, G., Nolen, W., Kupka, R., Grunze, H., et al. (2013). More stressors prior to and during the course of bipolar illness in patients from the United States compared with the Netherlands and Germany. *Psychiatry Research*, 210, 880–886.

Quevedo, Y., Booij, L., Herrera, L., Hernández, C., & Jiménez, J. P. (2022). Potential epigenetic mechanisms in psychotherapy: a pilot study on DNA methylation and mentalization change in borderline personality disorder. *Frontiers in Human Neuroscience*, 16, 955005. doi: 10.3389/fnhum.2022.955005.

Radtke, K. M., Ruf, M., Gunter, H. M., Dohrmann, K., Schauer, M., Meyer, A., & Elbert, T. (2011). Transgenerational impact of intimate partner violence on methylation in the promoter of the glucocorticoid receptor. *Translational Psychiatry*, 1(7), e21. https://doi.org/10.1038/tp.2011.21

Ríos, U., Moya, P. R., Urrejola, Ó., Hermosilla, J., Gonzalez, R., Munõz, P., et al. (2020). History of child abuse among patients with bipolar disorders. *Revista Médica de Chile*, 148, 204–210. doi: 10.4067/s0034-98872020000200204.

Romero, S., Birmaher, B., Axelson, D., et al. (2009). Prevalence and correlates of physical and sexual abuse in children and adolescents with bipolar disorder. *Journal of Affective Disorders*, 112, 144–150.

Rossi, J. L., Jiménez, J. P., Barros, P., Assar, R., Jaramillo, K., Herrera, L., et al. (2019). Depressive symptomatology and psychological well-being among Chilean university students. *Revista Médica de Chile*, 147, 579–588.

Slavich, G. M., & Cole, S. W. (2013). The emerging field of human social genomics. *Clinical Psychological Science*, 1(3), 331–348.

Teicher, M. H., Samson, J. A., Anderson, C. M., & Ohashi, K. (2016). The effects of childhood maltreatment on brain structure, function and connectivity. *Nature Reviews Neuroscience*, 17(10), 652–666. https://doi.org/10.1038/nrn.2016.111.

Thomas, P., Melchior, M., & Barnes, P. J. (2018). Glucocorticoid receptor gene methylation and the cortisol stress response in borderline personality disorder. *Translational Psychiatry*, 8(1), 55. doi: 10.1038/s41398-018-0107-7.

van IJzendoorn, M. H., Caspers, K., Bakermans-Kranenburg, M. J., Beach, S. R., & Philibert, R. (2010). Methylation matters: interaction between methylation density and serotonin transporter genotype predicts unresolved loss or trauma. *Biological Psychiatry*, 68(5), 405–407. https://doi.org/10.1016/j.biopsych.2010.05.008.

Zannas, A. S. (2016). Epigenetic programming of stress responses through variations in DNA methylation: life at the interface between a dynamic environment and a fixed genome. *Dialogues in Clinical Neuroscience*, 18(3), 353–363.

# 5 Diagnosis of personality organization – toward the evaluation of severity and change

*Stephan Doering*

## The efficacy research dilemma

During the last few decades of the 20th century, psychopharmacological treatments gained an enormous influence on psychiatry. They promised quick and cheap recovery to almost every patient. New generations of more effective substances with less side effects fueled the expectation of a complete control over mental disorders that, of course, were regarded as predominantly caused by brain malfunctioning. Moreover, pharmaceutic companies due to their financial power were able to afford huge randomized-controlled trials demonstrating the efficacy of their products, which in many cases included huge budgets for opinion leaders and their (university) departments.

No wonder that the classification systems of ICD-10 (World Health Organization 1992) and Diagnostic and Statistical Manual of Mental Disorders – DSMIV (American Psychiatric Association 1994) – that were created by opinion leaders in the field of psychiatry – employed a phenomenological and descriptive approach to diagnosis. That means diagnoses are solely based on symptoms and explicitly exclude any assumption on underlying (unconscious) etiological processes or aspects of personality and personality functioning. Only the visible tip of the iceberg seemed to be relevant for the assessment – which perfectly makes sense, if one focuses on the use of medication, which usually changes symptoms, but not personality or internalized object relations.

Under the influence of this zeitgeist, the Division 12 Task Force on Promotion and Dissemination of Psychological Procedures of the American Psychological Association resumed its work with the aim to defend psychotherapy against the overwhelming predominance of biological treatments in psychiatry. In an attempt to defeat pharmacology with its own weapons, the Task Force developed criteria for empirically-validated treatments (Chambless et al. 1998) (Table 5.1).

With slight modifications (Tolin et al. 2015), these criteria are still in effect until today. A website lists all psychological treatments with published evidence of efficacy (https://div12.org/psychological-treatments/). Interestingly, the large series of single case studies has not prevailed.

DOI: 10.4324/9781032651934-7

*Table 5.1* Criteria for Empirically-Validated Treatments (From Chambless et al. 1998, p. 4)

---

Well-Established Treatments

I. At least two good between-group design experiments demonstrating efficacy in one or more of the following ways:
   A. Superior (statistically significantly so) to pill or psychological placebo or to another treatment.
   B. Equivalent to an already established treatment in experiments with adequate sample sizes.

Or

II. A large series of single case design experiments (n>9) demonstrating efficacy. These experiments must have:
   C. Used good experimental designs and
   D. Compared the intervention to another treatment as in IA.

Further criteria for both I and II:

III. Experiments must be conducted with treatment manuals.
IV. Characteristics of the client samples must be clearly specified.
V. Effects must have been demonstrated by at least two different investigators or investigating teams.

Probably efficacious treatments

I. Two experiments showing the treatment is superior (statistically significantly so) to a waiting-list control group.

Or

II. One or more experiments meeting the Well-Established Treatment Criteria IA or IB, III, and IV, but not V.

Or

III. A small series of single case design experiments (n ≥ 3) otherwise meeting Well-Established Treatment.

---

Since the aim was to compare psychotherapy with medication, the outcome criteria were already determined by pharmacological studies as well as ICD-10 and DSM-IV, namely symptom change like reduced depression or anxiety in patients with depression or anxiety disorders. As a consequence, this development caused somewhat unfair competition from the beginning, since it implicitly favored behaviorally-oriented treatments that aim at symptom change over psychoanalysis. The goals of psychoanalysis have for a long time been a matter of controversy: Should psychoanalysis have any goals? If so, what should be its goals? Sigmund Freud gave some hints when he wrote in *Freud's Psycho-Analytic Procedure* (1904):

> Just as health and sickness are not different from each other in essence but are only separated by a quantitative line of quantification which can be determined in practice, so the aim of the treatment will never be anything else but the practical recovery of the patient, the restoration of his ability to lead an active life and of his capacity for enjoyment.

and in *The New Introductory Lectures on Psycho-Analysis* (1933), he phrased the famous "Where id was ego shall be".

A contemporary attempt to rephrase Freud's ideas could be the following:

The primary aim of psychoanalysis is personality change/maturation, awareness of the self and others (mentalization), and an increase of degrees of freedom in adapting to oneself and the social world – rather than mere symptom reduction.

Thus, psychoanalysis needs different research paradigms/dimensions of outcome. The direct competition with behaviorally oriented psychotherapies using symptoms as primary outcome measures tends to be unfavorable for psychoanalysis since most of the former tend to be shorter, quicker, and cheaper than psychoanalysis when it comes to symptom change, particularly in the absence of personality pathology.

As a consequence, a feasible demonstration of efficacy of psychoanalysis should include an assessment of changes in the patients' "ability to lead an active life and of his capacity for enjoyment", which has most frequently been translated into "capacity for love and work".

## Conceptualization of ego functions/personality organization

We can find conceptualizations of the capacity for love and work already in the early psychoanalytic concept of ego functions, e.g., Anna Freud's *The Ego and the Mechanisms of Defense* (1936) and Heinz Hartmann's *Ego Psychology and the Problem of Adaptation* (1939). These early ego-psychological conceptualizations promote the idea that one of the essential tasks of the ego is adaptation to external reality, stress, relationships, and occupational life. Besides ego psychology, it was object relations theory that contributed considerably to the conceptualization of the capacity for love and work. Otto Kernberg developed his model of personality organization as early as 1975, when he presented the trials of identity diffusion and primitive defensive operations with essential preservation of reality testing (p. 161). As we will see below, in his later work, he included primitive aggression, superego integration, and quality of object relations into his model of personality organization.

Among others, these psychoanalytic concepts paved the way for the recent development in mainstream psychiatry to make the impairment of personality functioning an essential criterion for the diagnosis of a personality disorder. This can be found in DSM-5 (American Psychiatric Association 2013, p. 761) as well as in ICD-11 (see: https://gcp.network/groupings/personality-disorders-and-related-traits/).

As will be discussed below, psychoanalytic treatment has already shown to be efficacious to improve personality functioning or organization (Doering et al. 2010), which is in line with the assumption that psychoanalysis can facilitate personality change and, thus, foster the capacity for love and work. To achieve these goals, longer treatments are more necessary than for mere symptom reduction, however, it can be assumed that symptom reduction in patients with low levels of personality organization takes considerably more time than in neurotic patients. This is one reason for the fact that most of the studies on the efficacy of psychotherapy exclude patients with comorbid personality disorders, which results in highly selected patient samples with low generalizability of the study results.

As a consequence, empirical research on the efficacy of psychoanalysis, which is urgently needed for the "survival" of psychoanalysis in mental health care systems of many countries in the world, should always include changes in personality organization as a primary outcome criterion. Meanwhile, a variety of structured measures for the assessment of this domain are available and will be presented briefly here.

## Diagnostic interviews for the assessment of personality organization

Since the early 1980s, a number of instruments emerged from psychoanalytic research to assess personality organization, which most recently mounted into the development of the DSM-5 conceptualization of personality functioning and an interview for its assessment (see Table 5.2).

*Table 5.2* Interviews for the Assessment of Personality Organization

|  | *Year* | *Dimensions* | *Structure* |
|---|---|---|---|
| Hampstead Index | 1981 | 10 | Clinical interview |
| Structural Interview | 1981 | For clinical use, no scoring | Clinical interview |
| Scales of Psychological Capacities (SPC) | 1991 | 17 scales, 35 subdimensions | Clinical interview with structured aspects |
| Operationalized Psychodynamic Diagnosis (OPD-3) | 1996/2023 | 9 scales, 27 subdimensions | Clinical interview with structured aspects |
| Structured Interview of Personality Organization (STIPO-R) | 2003/2016 | 6 scales, 11 subdimensions | (Semi-)structured |
| Structured Clinical Interview for the DSM-5 Alternative Model for Personality Disorder (SCID-5-AMPD) | 2018 | S scales, 4 subdimensions | (Semi-)structured |
| Social Cognition and Object Relations Scale (SCORS) | 1995 | 8 scales | Clinical interview/ stories |
| Adult Attachment Interview (AAI) | 1985 | 5 attachment types | Semi-structured interview |

An early precursor of contemporary structured interviews is the *Hampstead Index* that was developed based on Anna Freud's ego psychological works at the Anna Freud Center in London (Anna Freud Center 1981). The Hampstead Index as published in 1981 comprises ten dimensions (p. 218 f.):

1  General Case Material
2  Ego
   a  Functions
   b  Anxiety
   c  Defenses
3  Affects
4  Instinctual
5  Object Relationships
6  Superego
7  Symptoms
8  Treatment Situation and Technique
9  Comments and Theme
10  Special Interests

The Hampstead Index was created to structure diagnostic and process material with the aim to allow for a complete psychoanalytic case formulation.

Probably most influential for the development of the diagnosis assessment of personality functioning/organization was Otto Kernberg's *Structural Interview* (1981, 1984). The unstructured clinical interview aims at a structural diagnosis by focusing on the above-mentioned dimensions of Kernberg's object relational model. The interviewer's attitude is more active and structuring than in a psychoanalytic initial interview. An emphasis is on the elucidation of the patient's external reality, particularly object relations and occupational situation. Moreover, for the first time, the Structural Interview introduces the technique of asking for a detailed description of the self as well as a significant object, a tool that has been adopted by many interviews since then. However, the Structural Interview is not suited for research purposes, since it does not allow for a reliable quantification of personality organization and an assessment of change.

The first diagnostic interview that was developed for the assessment of structural change in psychotherapy research was Robert Wallerstein's *Scales of Psychological Capacities (SPC)* (Wallerstein 1991; de Witt et al. 1999). Seventeen scales that cover 35 subdimensions altogether are assigned to the two domains of self-capacities and relationship capacities (Table 5.3).

The German Task Force Operationalized Psychodynamic Diagnosis (OPD) published the first edition of a comprehensive diagnostic instrument in 1996. The first two editions comprised five axes (Task Force OPD 2008) that were recently reduced to four axes in the third edition, OPD-3 (Arbeitskreis OPD 2023). One of the four axes is the structure axis for the assessment of personality structure. This axis contains five domains with 27 facets (Table 5.4).

*Table 5.3* SPC (de Witt et al. 1999, p. 465 f.)

| Self-Capacities | Relationship Capacities |
| --- | --- |
| Hope | Empathy |
| Zest | Commitment |
| Responsibility | Reciprocity |
| Flexibility | Trust |
| Persistence | Assertion |
| Standards | Reliance |
| Affect | |
| Impulse | |
| Sexual | |
| Self-esteem | |
| Coherence | |

*Table 5.4* Structure Axis of the OPD-3 (Arbeitskreis OPD 2023, p. 193, translation S.D.)

| *Self* | *Object/Relationships* |
| --- | --- |
| *Self-perception* | *Object perception* |
| ST1.1 Self-reflection | ST1.4 Self-/object differentiation |
| ST1.2 Affect differentiation | ST1.5 Object-related affect differentiation |
| ST1.3 Identity | ST1.6 Integrated object perception |
| *Self-Regulation* | *Regulation of object relationship* |
| ST2.1 Impulse control | ST2.4 Protecting relationships |
| ST2.2 Affect tolerance | ST2.5 Anticipation |
| ST2.3 Self-worth regulation | ST2.6 Balancing of interests |
| *Defense* | |
| ST3.1 Options of life and experience | |
| ST3.2 Interpersonality | |
| ST3.3 Mechanisms | |
| *Internal Communication* | *Communication with the External World* |
| ST4.1 Experiencing affects and fantasies | ST4.4 Emotionally making contact |
| ST4.2 Joyful experience | ST4.5 Intimacy |
| ST4.3 Bodily self | ST4.6 Empathy |
| *Internal Objects* | *External Objects* |
| ST5.1 Internalization | ST5.4 Ability to make attachments |
| ST5.2 Use of introjects | ST5.5 Trust |
| ST5.3 Variable attachments | ST5.6 Severing attachments |

John Clarkin and colleagues developed the *Structured Interview of Personality Organization* (STIPO) that first came out in 2003 (Clarkin et al. 2003; Stern et al. 2010), meanwhile a revised version (STIPO-R; Clarkin et al. 2016) has been released (for download see https://istfp.org/publications/diagnostic-instruments/). The STIPO is rooted in the Kernberg's Structural Interview; it was created for research purposes to allow for a

*Table 5.5* Dimension of the STIPO – Revised Version
(STIPO-R; Clarkin et al. 2016)

---

Identity
  Capacity to invest
  Sense of self
  Representation of other
Object relations
  Interpersonal relationships
  Sex and intimacy
  Interpersonal investments in others
Lower-level "primitive" defenses
Higher-level defenses
Aggression
  Self-directed
  Other-directed
Moral values

---

reliable quantification of the dimensions of personality organization as conceptualized by Otto Kernberg. The STIPO-R comprises 55 questions that are read to the patient and the interviewer is supposed to use additional questions to probe until the answer is clear enough to be assessed on a three-point scale. Sum scores are calculated for six domains partly with subdomains (see Table 5.5). An overall assessment of the level of personality organization is made on a six-point scale (normal, neurotic 1 and 2, borderline 1, 2, and 3). In addition, 11 items are used to calculate a separate narcissism score that quantifies narcissistic pathology.

## Interviews focusing on object relations

A number of psychoanalytically informed interviews focus specifically on object relations, a core dimension of personality functioning that has been included into all of the before mentioned more comprehensive interviews. It has been shown repeatedly that the quality of object relations correlates highly with the overall score of personality organization (see, e.g., Stern et al. 2010; Doering et al. 2013).

The *Social Cognition and Object Relations Scale* (SCORS) was initially presented by Drew Westen (1995) as a Q-sort test. Stein and colleagues (2017) provided a *SCORS – Global Rating* (SCORS-G). The Scale is originally based on *the Thematic Apperception Test* (TAT; Morgan and Murray 1935). It uses stories and interview data to assess eight dimensions: (1) complexity of representations of people, (2) affective quality of representations, (3) capacity for emotional investment in relationships, (4) emotional investment in emotions and moral standards, (5) understanding of social causality, (6) experience and management of aggressive impulses, (7) self-esteem, (8) identity and coherence of self. Meanwhile, the SCORS is applied to a broad range of data, like, e.g., therapeutic sessions.

The *Adult Attachment Interview* (AAI) was developed by George, Kaplan, and Main (1985) and employs a linguistic approach to evaluate different attachment representations, a secure one and insecure ones (avoidant, preoccupied); in addition, unresolved trauma is diagnosed. Based on the AAI, Fonagy et al. (1998) designed the Reflective Functioning Scale (RF-Scale) that uses the answers to the AAI questions to assess what Fonagy later described as mentalization on a scale from "−1" to "9" (negative to high RF). Recently, the RF-Scale has been applied in a large variety of domains and data (see, e.g., Hartmann et al. 2015).

## Structural diagnosis arrived at the psychiatric mainstream

With the development of the DSM-5 (American Psychiatric Association 2013), the diagnosis of personality organization was introduced into the psychiatric mainstream. While it was planned to make so-called personality function, the primary diagnostic criterion for any personality disorder, in the last minute before the publication DSM-5, it was decided to keep the established diagnostic categories and ban the new approach into the appendix as an Alternative Model for Personality Disorders (AMPD) (p. 761). Nevertheless, the whole field focuses on the alternative model that has become the "main model" in the recently published *International Classification of Diseases – Eleventh Revision* (see Blüml and Doering 2021).

Both classifications combine an assessment of personality functioning with the assessment of an individual combination of personality traits and facets that are mainly based on the empirically derived big five factors of personality (Widiger 2017). The dimensions of personality functioning are almost identical and focus on two major domains, i.e., self and relationships. Table 5.6 shows the operationalization of these two domains with two subdomains each from the DSM-5 manual.

*Table 5.6* Elements of Personality Functioning of the DSM-5 AMPDs (American Psychiatric Association 2013, p. 762)

Self:

1 *Identity*: Experience of oneself as unique, with clear boundaries between self and others; stability of self-esteem and accuracy of self-appraisal; capacity for, and ability to regulate, a range of emotional experience.
2 *Self-direction*: Pursuit of coherent and meaningful short-term and life goals; utilization of constructive and prosocial internal standards of behavior; ability to self-reflect productively.

Interpersonal:

1 *Empathy*: Comprehension and appreciation of others' experiences and motivations; tolerance of differing perspectives; understanding the effects of one's own behavior on others.
2 *Intimacy*: Depth and duration of connection with others; desire and capacity for closeness; mutuality of regard reflected in interpersonal behavior.

The American Psychiatric Association has already provided a *Structured Clinical Interview for the DSM-5 AMPD* (SCID-5-AMPD; First et al. 2018). Like the diagnostic domains and criteria themselves, the interview is deeply rooted in its psychoanalytic precursors. The initial question "How would you describe yourself as a person?" has been taken from Otto Kernberg's *Structural Interview* (1981, 1984). From separate ratings of the four subdomains, an overall rating of personality functioning is made on a scale from "0 = little or no impairment" to "4 = extreme impairment".

## Questionnaires for the assessment of psychic structure (personality functioning)

For screening purposes, questionnaires have been developed to assess psychic structure or personality functioning, respectively. In 2001, the *Inventory of Personality Organization* (Clarkin et al. 2001; Lenzenweger et al. 2001) has been presented, a 56-item self-rating instrument that covers the domains reality testing, primitive defenses, and identity diffusion. A 95-item self-description questionnaire for the OPD structure axis was published in 2012 (Ehrenthal et al. 2012; Dinger et al. 2013). The instrument is available in English language. To assess the DSM-5 AMPD domains, an 80-item questionnaire (*Levels of Personality Functioning Scale, Self-rating*, LPFS-SR) has been published by Morey (2017).

In general, it can be stated that questionnaire can be used as screening tools and also for specific research questions, but they are not feasible for diagnosing personality organization or disorders. Clinical interviews are indispensable for a reliable diagnosis and the reveal diagnostic information that is needed for psychodynamic understanding and treatment planning, while questionnaires merely provide numbers.

## Use of the assessment of personality organization in psychotherapy studies

In light of our previous considerations, the turn toward a diagnostic assessment beyond symptoms represents a great opportunity for psychodynamic and psychoanalytic psychotherapy research. Finally, the outcome criteria for a treatment study can be chosen in accordance with the original concepts of treatment goals ("ability to lead an active life and of his capacity for enjoyment") and are not any longer restricted to symptom measures borrowed from psychopharmacological research paradigms.

A number of treatment studies already employed the above-mentioned instruments to determine change in personality organization as a documentation of efficacy of psychoanalytic treatments. The *Munich Psychotherapy Study* demonstrated the superiority of psychoanalysis over short-term psychodynamic psychotherapy and cognitive-behavioral therapy in depression using the SPC (Huber et al. 2012). Doering et al. (2010) used the

STIPO to demonstrate the efficacy of Transference-focused Psychotherapy (TFP; Yeomans et al. 2015) in patients with borderline personality disorder. Leuzinger-Bohleber et al. (2019) used the OPD to demonstrate structural change in depression; psychoanalysis was significantly superior to cognitive behavioral treatment.

It is strongly recommended to use one of the above-mentioned instruments for the assessment of change and outcome in psychotherapy studies on psychoanalysis. If possible, interviews should be employed since their sensitivity to change has already been demonstrated in large outcome studies. Finally, it should not be avoided to use the SCID-5-AMPD and/or the LPFS-SF to connect the results directly to mainstream psychiatric research and allow for comparisons and meta-analyses.

## References

American Psychiatric Association (1994). *Diagnostic and Statistical Manual of Mental Disorders*, Fourth Edition, DSM-IV. Washington, DC: American Psychiatric Press.

American Psychiatric Association (2013). *Diagnostic and Statistical Manual of Mental Disorders*, Fifth Edition, DSM-5. Washington, DC: American Psychiatric Press.

Anna Freud Center (1981). The Hampstead Index. *The Bulletin of the Anna Freud Center* 4:217–220.

Arbeitskreis OPD (2023). *OPD-3 - Operationalisierte Psychodynamische Diagnostik Das Manual für Diagnostik und Therapieplanung*. Göttingen: Hogrefe.

Blüml V, Doering S (2021). ICD-11 Personality Disorders: A Psychodynamic Perspective on Personality Functioning. *Frontiers in Psychiatry* 12:654026.

Chambless DL, Baker MJ, Baucom DH, Beutler LE, Calhoun KS, Crits-Christoph P, Daiuto A, De Rubeis R, Detweiler J, Haage DAF, Bennett Johnson S, McCurry S, Mueser KT, Poper KS, Sanderson WC, Shoham V, Stickle T, Williams DA, Woody SR (1998). An Update on Empirically Validated Therapies II. *The Clinical Psychologist* 51(1):5–18.

Clarkin JF, Caligor E, Stern B, Kernberg OF (2003). *Structured Interview of Personality Organization (STIPO)*. New York: Weill Medical College of Cornell University.

Clarkin JF, Caligor E, Stern BL, Kernberg OF (2016). *Structured Interview of Personality Organization–Revised (STIPO-R)*. New York: Weill Medical College of Cornell University.

Clarkin JF, Foelsch PA, Kernberg OF (2001). *The Inventory of Personality Organization*. New York: Weill Medical College of Cornell University.

de Witt KN, Milbrath C, Wallerstein RS (1999). Scales of Psychological Capacities: Support for a Measure of Structural Change. *Psychoanalysis and Contemporary Thought* 22:453–480.

Dinger U, Schauenburg H, Hörz S, Rentrop M, Komo-Lang M, Klinkerfuß M, Köhling J, Grande T, Ehrenthal JC (2013). Self-Report and Observer Ratings of Personality Functioning: A Study of the OPD System. *Journal of Personality Assessment* 96(2):220–225.

Doering S, Burgmer M, Heuft G, Menke D, Bäumer B, Lübking M, Feldmann M, Hörz S, Schneider G (2013). Reliability and Validity of the German Version of the Structured Interview of Personality Organization (STIPO). BMC Psychiatry 13:210.

Doering S, Hörz S, Rentrop M, Fischer-Kern M, Schuster P, Benecke C, Buchheim A, Martius P, Buchheim P (2010). Transference-Focused Psychotherapy v. Treatment by Community Psychotherapists for Borderline Personality Disorder: Randomised Controlled Trial. *British Journal of Psychiatry* 196:389–395.

Ehrenthal JC, Dinger U, Horsch L, Komo-Lang M, Klinkerfuss M, Grande T, Schauenburg H (2012). The OPD Structure Questionnaire (OPD-SQ): First Results on Reliability and Validity. *Psychotherapie, Psychosomatik, Medizinische Psychologie* 62(1):25–32.

First MB, Skodol AE, Bender DS, Oldham JM (2018). *Structured Clinical Interview for the DSM-5 Alternative Model for Personality Disorders (SCID-5-AMPD)*. Arlington, VA: American Psychiatric Publishing.

Fonagy P, Target M, Steele H, Steele M (1998). *Reflective-Functioning Manual*, Version 5, for application to Adult Attachment Interviews. London: Psychoanalysis Unit, University College London.

Freud, A (1936). *The Ego and the Mechanisms of Defense*. Madison, CT: International Universities Press, 1966.

Freud, S. (1904). *Freud's Psycho-analytic Procedure*, Standard Edition 7. London: Hogarth Press, 1953, pp. 249–254.

Freud, S. (1933). New Introductory Lectures on Psycho-Analysis, Standard Edition, Vol. 22. London: Hogarth Press, 1964.

George C, Kaplan N, Main M (1985). *The Adult Attachment Interview*. Berkeley: Department of Psychology, University of California at Berkeley.

Hartmann H (1939). *Ego Psychology and the Problem of Adaptation*. Madison, CT: International Universities Press, 1958.

Hartmann LK, Neubert V, Läzer KL, Ackermann P, Schreiber M, Fischmann T, Leuzinger-Bohleber M (2015). Mentalization and the Impact of Psychoanalytic Case Supervision. *Journal of the American Psychoanalytic Association* 63(3):NP20–NP22.

Huber D, Henrich G, Gastner J, Klug G (2012). Must All Have Prizes? The Munich Psychotherapy Study. In: Levy R, Ablon J, Kächele H (eds.) *Psychodynamic Psychotherapy Research*. Totowa, NJ: Current Clinical Psychiatry, Humana Press, 51–69.

Kernberg OF (1975). *Borderline Conditions and Pathological Narcissism*. Oxford: Jason Aronson.

Kernberg OF (1981). Structural Interviewing. *Psychiatric Clinics of North America* 4(1):169–195.

Kernberg OF (1984). *Severe Personality Disorders: Psychotherapeutic Strategies*. New Haven, CT: Yale University Press.

Lenzenweger MF, Clarkin JF, Kernberg OF, Foelsch PA (2001). The Inventory of Personality Organization: Psychometric Properties, Factorial Composition, and Criterion Relations with Affect, Aggressive Dyscontrol, Psychosis Proneness, and Self-Domains in a Nonclinical Sample. *Psychological Assessment* 13:577–591.

Leuzinger-Bohleber M, Kaufhold J, Kallenbach L, Negele A, Ernst M, Keller W, Fiedler G, Hautzinger M, Bahrke U, Beutel M (2019). How to Measure Sustained Psychic Transformations in Long-Term Treatments of Chronically Depressed Patients: Symptomatic and Structural Changes in the LAC Depression Study of the Outcome of Cognitive-Behavioural and Psychoanalytic Long-Term Treatments. International Journal of Psychoanalysis 100(1):99–127.

Morey LC (2017). Development and Initial Evaluation of a Self-Report Form of the DSM-5 Level of Personality Functioning Scale. *Psychological Assessment* 29:1302–1308.

Morgan CD, Murray HA (1935). A Method for Investigating Fantasies: The Thematic Apperception Test. *Archives of Neurology and Psychiatry* 34(2):289–306.

Stein MB, Slavin-Mulford J (2017). *The Social Cognition and Object Relations Scale-Global Rating Method (SCORS-G): A Comprehensive Guide for Clinicians and Researchers*. London: Routledge.

Stern BL, Caligor E, Clarkin JF, Critchfield KL, Horz S, MacCornack V, Lenzenweger MF, Kernberg OF (2010). Structured Interview of Personality Organization (STIPO): Preliminary Psychometrics in a Clinical Sample. *Journal of Personality Assessment* 92:35–44.

Task Force OPD (2008). *Operationalized Psychodynamic Diagnosis – OPD-2*. Bern: Huber.

Tolin DF, Mckay D, Forman EM, Klonsky ED, Thombs BD (2015). Empirically Supported Treatment: Recommendations for a New Model. *Clinical Psychology: Science and Practice* 22(4):317–338.

Wallerstein RS (1991). Assessment of Structural Change in Psychoanalytic Therapy and Research. In: Shapiro T (ed.) *The Concept of Structure in Psychoanalysis*. Madison, CT: International Universities Press, pp. 241–261.

Westen D (1995). *Social Cognition and Object Relations Scale: Q-sort for Projective Stories (SCORS-Q)*. Cambridge, MA: Department of Psychiatry, The Cambridge Hospital and Harvard Medical School.

Widiger TA (ed.) (2017). *The Oxford Handbook of the Five Factor Model*. New York: Oxford University Press.

World Health Organization (1992). *The ICD-10 Classification of Mental and Behavioural Disorders*. Geneva: World Health Organization.

World Health Organization (2023). *The ICD-11 Classification of Diseases. 11ᵗʰ Revision. ICD-11*. Geneva: World Health Organization. Online: https://icd.who.int/en.

Yeomans F, Clarkin JF, Kernberg OF, Kernberg OF (2015). *Transference-Focused Psychotherapy for Borderline Personality Disorder: A Clinical Guide*. Arlington, VA: American Psychiatric Publishing.

# 6 Group analytic psychotherapy. An effective treatment?

*Steinar Lorentzen*

## Introduction

Psychoanalytic therapies are important elements in public mental health services, whether they are offered to individual patients, groups, or in other formats. Meta-analyses show that group psychotherapy, *in general*, is effective for a variety of psychological disorders (Burlingame & Strauss, 2021). Comparisons between individual and group therapies gave similar results as to therapy acceptance, symptomatic improvement, and drop-out rates between the two formats (Burlingame et al., 2016). The efficacy of psychodynamic and group-analytic psychotherapies has, however, only been studied in a few randomized trials. One reason for the scarcity of studies may be that methodological challenges are greater in psychodynamic research, which aim at studying phenomena affected by unconscious forces (see Introduction to this volume).

Despite scarcity of empirical evidence on groups, results from many studies on individual psychodynamic psychotherapy also are valid for group psychotherapy. Furthermore, research results from group therapies of different theoretical orientations may also be valid for psychodynamic group psychotherapy, for example, the significance of leadership, group structure, cohesion, and other therapeutic factors (Yalom & Leszcz, 2020).

This chapter will demonstrate the *effectiveness* and *efficacy* of *group-analytic psychotherapy*, which is probably the most used psychodynamic group approach in Europe. It was developed by S. H. Foulkes (1898–1976), a German–Jewish psychiatrist and psychoanalyst, in the late 1930s. Two central concepts for understanding and conceptualizing the individual in group therapy are *foundation matrix* and *dynamic matrix*, respectively. Foundation matrix is based on the fact that all human beings have a biological and cultural background and have been born into and socialized in a family. This common fate leads to a connectedness between humans, and to a need for communication and a language, all being factors of vital importance for people to understand each other. The dynamic matrix is a created and potentially intimate network developed by the members of the therapy group. It is defined as "a hypothetical network of communications and relationships"

DOI: 10.4324/9781032651934-8

or "the network of all individual mental processes, the psychological medium in which they meet, communicate and interact" (Foulkes, 1977).

Foulkes was also concerned with how a group could devote itself to a "free-floating discussion" in line with the "free associations" seen in psychoanalysis, believing that the therapist's laid back, pending attitude would elicit free associations having cues to latent themes indicative of individual and collective processes in the group as a whole. He also recommended that therapists should tone down their authority, thus mobilizing the treatment resources of individual members. For further information on his theories, the reader is referred to Foulkes' own writings or secondary literature (Barwick & Weegmann, 2018; Behr & Hearst, 2005; Foulkes, 1984, 1986; Foulkes & Anthony, 1984; Lorentzen, 2022; Pines, 1983, 1994; Schlapobersky, 2016).

This chapter presents research evidence for group analysis and analytic/dynamic group psychotherapy and points to the urgent need for doing more research. Another aim is to demonstrate that research on long-term group (LTG) and short-term group (STG) analytic therapies following high research standards is feasible. This implies e.g., developing a treatment manual, randomization of patients, check of therapist adherence and competence, and the application of relevant outcome measures that catch changes in mental distress as well as dysfunctional aspects of personality structure.

## Summary of results from three different sources of research

Excerpts from a systematic review of analytic/dynamic group psychotherapy commissioned by Institute of Group Analysis/Group-Analytic Society, London, are briefly summarized in the first step (Blackmore et al., 2012, see section "A review of group analysis and analytic/dynamic group psychotherapy"). The review was intended to strengthen the position of psychodynamic therapies within the National Health Services of UK. In the second step, research from the author's own research group is described; *one observational study* and *one randomized clinical trial* (RCT). This research is one of very few that have produced quantitative group-analytic research since the previously mentioned review was done (see sections "The effectiveness of LTG analysis: an observational study" and "A randomized clinical trial; short- vs. long-term group-analytic therapy"). Finally, a new "Focused Group-Analytic Psychotherapy" (Lorentzen, 2022) is presented, illustrating how a theoretical coherence between patient factors assessed at pre-therapy, treatment guidelines, and outcome and process measures can be implemented (section "Focused group analytic psychotherapy").

### *A review of group analysis and analytic/dynamic group psychotherapy*

Professionals from Centre for Psychological Services, Sheffield University, searched central databases for group-analytic and analytic/dynamic group studies published in English during the years 2001–2008 which included a control or comparison group. Thirty-four primary studies and 19 reviews, the last intending to cover studies carried out before 2001, were located.

Five of the primary studies were *RCTs* that provided evidence for the efficacy of group therapy on a range of clinical problems, but there was no evidence that benefits were specific to psychodynamic/analytic groups. One of the RCTs (Blay et al., 2002) found a positive effect of brief psychodynamic group therapy compared to usual care. Another study found a positive effect of modified group analysis, but this was smaller than in the control, a systemic group therapy (Lau & Kristensen, 2007). Three studies did not find any significant differences between psychodynamic and other active group treatments (Lanza et al., 2002; Piper et al., 2001; Tasca et al., 2006). The trials ranged from poor to good methodological quality.

There were five case-control studies using a matched or waitlist comparison group. Several of these provided good support for the use of group psychotherapy in a variety of conditions. In two studies of partially hospitalized patients, it was impossible to extract data separately for the effects of individual and group psychotherapies. The rest of the studies, including several made on long-term therapies, were observational, the results suggesting significant benefits of psychodynamic group psychotherapy. However, it is not possible to attribute changes to the group intervention, as there were no control groups. One example of an observational study is presented below.

The 19 reviews, most covering studies before 2001, included analytic group therapy amongst many other interventions. The studies confirmed that group therapies in general are more effective than waitlist or standard care control. Only one review summarized both outcome and process research in group-analytic treatment, acknowledging the problem of differentiating between group-analytic and other psychodynamic studies (Lorentzen, 2006).

*Predictors and moderators*

Predictors alter treatment response irrespective of treatment condition, whereas moderators differentially influence whether someone is likely to benefit from a particular type of treatment. Several studies examined *predictors*, finding, e.g., that someone is likely to benefit from a particular form of treatment depending on sociodemographic characteristics such as gender, age, or personal characteristics such as attachment style or psychological mindedness. One study stressed that predictors of change in LTGs are likely to be different from those for STGs (Lorentzen & Høglend, 2004).

Eleven studies examined *moderators*, evidence suggesting important effects of age, gender, self-efficacy, treatment duration, and psychological mindedness on clinical outcomes. These effects have been reported for specific patient groups and may not generalize to others. Effects may also be moderated by group cohesion and individual factors, e.g., men may do less well in mixed sex groups where they are in minority, because they are unable to resolve interpersonal issues (Ogrodniczuk, 2006).

### The effectiveness of long-term group analysis: an observational study

The author started, in the late 1980s, a study of patients treated in three slow-open groups in a private specialist practice and collected data systematically from 69 patients. The aims were to study therapy *effectiveness*, *predictors* of change, and the relationship between *process* and *outcome*. The therapist interviewed the patients before and after therapy. An independent evaluator was included at follow-up, one year after termination. Patients were diagnosed with anxiety and depressive disorders (Diagnostic and Statistical Manual, version 3-Revised; DSM-3-R). 68% had a diagnosis of personality disorder (PD; Cluster B, C or mixed). About 54% were women. Patients had a mean age of 36 years. The therapist assessed the patients' psychosocial functioning. The patients gave self-reports of symptoms and interpersonal problems. Results: Mean time in therapy was 32.5 months (range six months to eight years). Only two patients dropped out of therapy. Effect-sizes of the changes after therapy were moderate to large. Patients continued to change until follow-up, one year later, when 61%–86% were clinically significantly improved/recovered on all outcome measures (Lorentzen et al., 2002). Predictors of outcome and the relationship between process and outcome associations are discussed in Lorentzen and Høglend (2004, 2005) and Lorentzen et al. (2004).

Interaction effects between patient aspects and therapy length were calculated, indicating that longer therapies were desirable for patients with *a higher initial degree of* depression, more general symptomatic distress, rating themselves higher on "interpersonal sensitivity", who were diagnosed with a more severe personality disorder (Cluster B), or were characterized as "less assertive", more "exploitable", or more "intrusive", based on the interpersonal circumplex (see Inventory of Interpersonal problems under section "Focused group analytic psychotherapy") (Lorentzen & Høglend, 2008). To further test out the significance of treatment duration with an improved design, a multi-site RCT was planned (Lorentzen et al., 2013).

### A randomized clinical trial; short- vs. long-term group-analytic therapy

This is the first RCT comparing the outcomes of STG and LTG analytic psychotherapies, within the same study. A detailed research protocol and treatment manuals were produced (Lorentzen, 2014). Study sites and experienced therapists were invited in and pre-trained in the relevant therapies.

One hundred and sixty-seven patients with mixed diagnoses (primarily anxiety and depressive disorders, 45% with a diagnosis of one or more PDs) were randomized to the two therapies, consisting of 20 or 80 weekly, 90-minute sessions. There were 18 closed groups and nine therapists, all conducting a group of each type.

Patients were interviewed by an independent evaluator before therapy and three years later, and symptoms and interpersonal problems (self-reports), and psychosocial functioning (observer-rated) were selected as outcome variables. Self-reports were collected at seven time-points during the seven-year study period. Psychosocial functioning was rated at pre-therapy and at three-year follow-up. Repeated measures of process were also collected, and intent-to treat-analyses with linear mixed models were used. Therapy sessions were audio-taped, and treatment fidelity was evaluated.

*Results*

Potential differences in outcomes for patients treated in short-term group (STG) and long-term group (LTG) were analyzed for "the typical patient" (average across the sub-samples), for patients *with* a diagnosis of personality disorders, and finally, for patients *without* personality disorders.

*The typical patient*

Patients in both groups made significant gains, but no significant differences could be detected for outcome between the short- and long-therapy groups at any time-point, up to three years, except that short-term therapy was superior to long-term therapy in symptomatic improvement at six months (Lorentzen et al., 2013). After the termination of the long-term therapy, patients continued to improve for the next four years and had a *delayed effect* from the end of therapy to the seven-year follow-up. The patients in short-term therapy *maintained* the improvement obtained by the end of therapy, also at seven-year follow-up. The effect-sizes of differences between the therapies from three to seven years follow-up in symptoms and interpersonal problems were small and moderate, respectively, in favor of long-term therapy (Lorentzen et al., 2015a).

There were also differences in changes in *self-perception* and in how patients perceived changes within eight interpersonal domains of interpersonal problems between the two treatments, and interested readers are referred to Lorentzen et al. (2015b) and Fjeldstad et al. (2017). Most important differences in *cohesion-outcome associations* between short- and long-term therapies were that cohesion is an important predictor of outcomes (symptoms and interpersonal problems) in the short-term therapy, but not in the LTGs (Lorentzen et al., 2018).

*Patients with and without a personality disorder*

As hypothesized, PD patients improved significantly more on all outcome variables in LTG compared to STG, during the first three years. The effect-sizes of the differences in outcomes were medium. Inspection of the data showed, however, that patients with PDs changed *to equal degree* in the two therapies on both symptomatic and interpersonal distress, during the *first six* months. For patients *without* PD, the rate of change was *similar* across three years on all outcome variables. However, the rate of change in symptoms and interpersonal problems was *higher in STG*, during the first six months. Patients without PD did not get any additional gain from LTG (Lorentzen et al., 2015c).

When the data from the seven-year follow-up was added, it turned out that patients with PD changed significantly more in the LTG compared to the STGs from six months to seven years. However, patients without personality disorder responded equally in the two treatments over the last 6.5 years (Fjeldstad et al., 2016).

*Focused group-analytic psychotherapy*

Based on research and clinical experience, the author has formulated a new therapy called "Focused Group Analytic Psychotherapy" (FGAP; Lorentzen, 2022). This is a time-limited therapy, suitable for patients with a medium to high level of personality organization (PO). FGAP takes place in a closed group with seven to eight patients and one to two therapists and consists of twenty weekly sessions, each lasting for 90 minutes. The goal is to initiate a change process in each patient that can continue after termination.

While Foulkes was trained and oriented in ego-psychology, later group-analysts have put more weight on self-psychology, object-relations theory, and interpersonal theory, which underline the person's need for connectedness to others more strongly. FGAP shares Foulkes' understanding of the group as a whole, as a gestalt comprised of all its members, constituting more than the sum of what each member brings into the group (foundation-matrix). In addition, the group develops its own history through multilateral interactions and communications between members (dynamic matrix). FGAP also shares the idea that all communications in the group are *transpersonal*, affecting all members on a conscious or unconscious level. Likewise, each individual will influence the other members and the group, and thus, both individuals and the group as a whole have a marked impact via unconscious processes (Hopper, 2003).

Kernberg's object relations theory, having a central role in FGAP, integrates ideas of psychoanalytic drive and structural theory with object-relations and self-theory. His initial theories of how PO could be characterized as neurotic, borderline, or psychotic originated with his work on serious personality disorders (Kernberg, 1975, 1980, 1984), later developed into a dimensional system for evaluating PO *in general*, based on the assessment of developmental level of *structural elements* like identity, object relations, maturity of defenses, aggression tolerance/control, and moral values (Caligor et al., 2018). The theory explains how a person develops in relation to early significant others and gradually builds an internal world of *representations* that influence self-perception, attachment style, relational capacity, cognition, affects, and overt behavior.

Four basic premises constitute *anchors* in the frame of the FGAP. *First*, it is a *time-limited* therapy, meaning that patients must be motivated and have the resources to use feedback in order to change relatively quickly. They should settle for limited, circumscribed goals, that can be formulated as a focus for the therapy, and preparation before therapy may speed up the process. A *second point* is that FGAP takes place within a psychoanalytic theoretical framework. This implies that personality structures, unconscious motivation, level of PO, defenses, and resistance become central, as does interconnectedness, i.e., the relationships to others and self. Consequently, a treatment focus should have support in a psychodynamic case formulation, drawing connections between internal conflicts, interpersonal problems, and defenses. A *third point* is that FGAP is oriented toward the *individual*, and the aim is to alleviate *suffering* caused by psychological problems and/or mental disorders. This is done by making the patients *aware* of repetitive dysfunctional ways of *acting* or *feeling* in relation to others or self and help them to better understand how these behaviors have impact on others and the self, and how they are triggered and maintained. The *final aspect* is *the group* itself, which represents *the medium of change* via the dynamic matrix and therapeutic factors, facilitated by a relatively active and directive therapist, who works for the development of a group-analytic treatment culture. The therapists have the ultimate responsibility for balancing supportive and more evocative forces in the group, reminding patients of their therapy foci, keeping the process in the here-and-now, and working from the manifest toward the latent, i.e., helping the group members to obtain self-understanding.

*Evaluation*

In order to make FGAP work, it is vital to have a thorough understanding of the patient's psychological functioning, starting with the evaluation of *the patients' level of PO*. Besides, a relevant *therapy focus* founded in a psychodynamic case formulation (hypothesis) should be negotiated with the patient. Furthermore, a self-report of the patients' *interpersonal circumplex* is needed, as well as a clinical diagnosis. All relevant information can be collected through clinical and psychodynamic interviews with emphasis on actual complaints and problems, when and how mental disorders started and developed, underlining the importance of the patients' developmental history, personality description, and information on close relationships over the years. Potential patterns of transference–countertransference can often be elicited from the patient's description of close relationships, and the interviewer could also include a psychodynamic section in the interviews, trying to tune into and explore aspects of "distortions" and test out hypotheses about connections between "there-and-then" and "here-and-now". During this procedure, the patients' ability to observe themselves and to mentalize can be evaluated.

*Level of personality organization*

Personal resources are an essential issue since patients in FGAP must endure the relatively structured framework of the therapy, entailing opening up early and disclosing vulnerable parts of themselves, taking feedback from others, and focusing on work in the here-and-now. Diagnosing level of PO requires training and experience, and no recipe for how to evaluate level of PO is included here. Caligor et al. (2018) give a detailed description of how five levels of PO, normal, neurotic, and high, middle, and low level of borderline PO can be described based on ratings of five (or more) domains of personality structure. These are identity (capacity to and satisfaction from investment in work/spare time. Sense of self and others), object relations (number of friends, quality, and stability of friendships), maturity of defenses (from sublimation, humor to idealizing/devaluating, splitting), aggression (tolerance/control, directed toward self or others), and moral values (more or less important in directing a person's actions). Clinical anchors are offered for rating each domain on a scale from 1 (normal) to 5 (severe pathology). A mean score of 1 to 5 represents the levels of PO. Patients with an average score of three or less (i.e., normal, neurotic, or high borderline levels of PO) will be most suitable for FGAP. The evidence for this view builds on ratings of numerous case stories of *group patients* using the clinical anchors mentioned.

Caligor et al.'s system is a clinical version of the Structured Interview for Personality Organization (STIPO-R; Clarkin et al., 2016). The interview and a scoring sheet are available at http://www.borderlinedisorders.com. It is also possible to use other structured interviews or standardized questionnaires for diagnosing the level of PO, like DSM-5, section III (American Psychiatric Association, 2013), Operationalized Psychodynamic Diagnosis, version 2 (OPD-2; OPD Task Force, 2008), and Psychodynamic Diagnostic Manual, version 2 (PDM-2; Lingiardi & McWilliams, 2017).

*Inventory of interpersonal problems*

This is a self-report of the patient's interpersonal problems, based on the *Inventory of Interpersonal Problems* (IIP-circumplex; Alden et al., 1990). The profile indicates how patients see themselves compared to others within the eight subscales of dominance, intrusiveness, overly nurturance, exploitability, non-assertiveness, social avoidance, coldness, and vindictiveness.

*Treatment focus*

The patients should have a treatment focus, for example, a dysfunctional interpersonal pattern or a cluster of symptoms, with roots in a psychodynamic case formulation/hypothesis, linking vulnerability in the personality with stressors and clinical resultants (dysfunctional personality traits/

symptoms) (Cabaniss, 2013). Aspects of the IIP profile or one or more internal conflicts may also be part of the focus.

More resourceful patients may be treated in FGAP despite a moderate tendency to acting out, if the patient has a capacity to explore the impulsive behavior. It may even be selected as *the* main focus for the therapy. The initial evaluation also includes *a clinical diagnosis* (DSM-V).

## Final comments and recommendations

The Sheffield review presented in this chapter describes several *limitations* in the field of analytic/psychodynamic group research and offers *recommendations* for improvement (Blackmore et al., 2012). Many of the critical remarks as well as recommendations for future research are seconded by this author. It has, for example, been difficult to retrieve research results because many existing studies lack structured abstracts, key words, and clearly defined terminology in describing analytic/dynamic group psychotherapy. Another problem is the use of a variety of different outcome measures which in addition to showing great variations in methodological quality across studies also make comparisons of results difficult. The main problem within this field, however, is the scarcity of high-quality research done, resulting in a very low number of RCTs, and the fact that almost no observational studies are replicated. There is thus an urgent need for more research, both RCTs and practice-based evidence for the effectiveness of psychodynamic group psychotherapies. It seems important to study what kind of patients will be most likely to benefit from psychodynamic groups, by doing a head-to-head comparisons between psychodynamic and cognitive behavioral group therapies. It could also be of great interest to do comparative studies between psychodynamic therapies of different formats (individual and group) and integrate questions on predictors and moderators with those on mechanisms of change. In that way, more personalized psychodynamic knowledge could be generated, helping therapists to tailor various psychodynamic treatments to different populations of patients. Mediators (mechanisms of change) are factors that bring about change in symptoms. They must be shown themselves to change during therapy, a change that must precede the change in symptoms. These conditions have been fulfilled in a few studies, indicating that relevant mediators of change in psychodynamic therapies can be increase in insight or self-understanding, change in maturity of defenses, increase in reflective functioning and mentalization, and decrease in rigidity of personality (Barber et al., 2021).

The idea of presenting the trial with *random allocation* of outpatients to group therapies of different durations here is to show that doing high-quality research is feasible. Another attempt of responding to *some of* the criticism raised by the Sheffield group is the construction of FGAP. A main idea with this therapy is to take personality structures seriously since analytic therapies aim at and leads to structural change. This is done by carefully assessing dimensions of personality structure before and after therapy. The model is partly adopted from the research lab of Clarkin et al. (2016), in their work with transference-focused (individual) psychotherapy. For more information on evaluation of personality pathology, see Chapters 1 (Clarkin, J. et al.) and 5 (Doering, S.). Another idea is to have a theoretical coherence between patient factors (structural aspects of personality), treatment guidelines (theory and concepts), and measures of process (cohesion/alliance) and outcome (personality dimensions, symptomatic/interpersonal distress). A final important point is to have an empirical basis for patient suitability for the therapy offered, which means in this case to only include patients with a normal, neurotic, or a high borderline level of PO.

## References

Alden, L.E., Wiggins, J.S., & Pincus, A.L. (1990). Construction of circumplex scales for the inventory of interpersonal problems. *Journal of Personality Assessment*, 55: 521–536.

American Psychiatric Association. (2013). *Diagnostic and Statistical Manual of Mental Disorders*. Washington, DC: American Psychiatric Association.

Barber, J.P., Muran, J.C., McCarthy, K.S., Keefe, J.R., & Zilcha-Mano, S. (2021). Research on Dynamic Therapies. In M. Barkham, W. Lutz, & L.G. Castonguay (Eds.) *Bergin and Garfield's Handbook of Psychotherapy and Behavior Change* (pp. 387–419). Hoboken, NJ: John Wiley.

Barwick, N., & Weegmann, M. (2018). *Group Therapy. A Group-Analytic Approach*. London and New York: Routledge.

Behr, H., & Hearst, L. (2005). *Group-Analytic Psychotherapy. A Meeting of Minds*. London and Philadelphia, PA: Whurr Publishers.

Blackmore, C., Tantam, D., Parry, G., & Chambers, E. (2012). Report on a Systematic Review of the Efficacy and Clinical Effectiveness of Group Analysis and Analytic/Dynamic Group Psychotherapy. *Group Analysis*, 45(1): 46–69.

Blay, S. L., Vel Fucks, J. S., Barruzi, M., Di Pietro, M. C., Gastal, F. L., Neto, A. M., De Souza, M. P, Glausiusz, L. R. U., & Dewey, M. (2002). Effectiveness of Time-Limited Psychotherapy for Minor Psychiatric Disorders: Randomized Controlled Trial Evaluating Immediate v. Long-Term Effects. *British Journal Psychiatry*, 180: 416–422.

Burlingame, G.M., Seebeck, J.D., Janis, R.A., & Whitcomb, K.E. (2016). Outcome Differences between Individual and Group Formats When Identical and Nonidentical Treatments, Patients, and Doses Are Compared: A 25-Year Meta-Analytic Perspective. *Psychotherapy*, 53(4): 446–461.

Burlingame, G.M., & Strauss, B. (2021). Efficacy of Small Group Treatments: Foundation for Evidence-Based Practice. In M. Barkham, W. Lutz, & L.G. Castonguay (Eds.) *Bergin and Garfield's Handbook of Psychotherapy and Behavior Change* (pp. 583–624). Hoboken, NJ: John Wiley.

Cabaniss, D.L. (2013). *Psychodynamic Formulation*. Chichester: John Wiley & Sons.

Caligor, E., Kernberg, O.F., Clarkin, J.F., & Yeoman, F.E. (2018). *Psychodynamic Therapy for Personality Pathology. Treating Self and Interpersonal Functioning*. Washington, DC: American Psychiatric Association.

Clarkin, J.F., Caligor, E., Stern, B.L., & Kernberg, O. (2016). The Structured Interview of Personality Organization: STIPO-R. Available at: www.borderlinedisorders.com.

Fjeldstad, A., Høglend, P.A., & Lorentzen, S. (2016). Presence of Personality Disorder Moderates the Long-Term Effects of Short-Term and Long-Term Psychodynamic Group Therapy: A 7-Year Follow-Up of a Randomized Clinical Trial. *Group Dynamics: Theory, Research, and Practice*, 20(4): 294–309.

Fjeldstad, A., Høglend, P.A., & Lorentzen, S. (2017). Patterns of Change in Interpersonal Problems during and After Short-Term and Long-Term Psychodynamic Therapy. *Psychotherapy Research*, 27(3–4): 350–361.

Foulkes, S.H. (1977). *Therapeutic Group Analysis*. New York: International University Press.

Foulkes, S.H. (1984). *Introduction to Group-Analytic Psychotherapy*. London: Maresfield Reprints.

Foulkes, S.H., & Anthony, E.J. (1984). *Group Psychotherapy. The Psychoanalytical Approach*. London: Karnac.

Foulkes, S.H. (1986). *Group Analytic Psychotherapy. Method and Principles*. London: Maresfield Library.

Hopper, E. (2003). *The Social Unconscious. Selected Papers*. London and Philadelphia, PA: Jessica Kingsley Publishers.

Kernberg, O.F. (1975). *Borderline Conditions and Pathological Nacissism*. New York: Jason Aronson.

Kernberg, O. (1980). *Internal World and External Reality. Object Relations Theory Applied*. New York and London: Jason Aronson.

Kernberg, O.F. (1984). *Severe Personality Disorders: Psychotherapeutic Strategies*. New Haven, CT and London: Yale University Press.

Lanza, M.L., Anderson, J., Boisvert, C.M., LeBlanc, A., Fardy, M., & Steel, B. (2002). Assaultive Behavior Intervention in the Veterans Administration: Psychodynamic Group Psychotherapy Compared to Cognitive Behavior Therapy. *Perspectives in Psychiatric Care*, 38: 89–97.

Lau, M., & Kristensen, E. (2007). Outcome of Systemic and Analytic Psychotherapy for Adult Women with History of Intrafamilial Childhood Sexual Abuse: A Randomized Controlled Study. *Acta Psychiatrica Scandinavica*, 116(2): 96–104.

Lingiardi, V., & McWilliams, N. (Eds.). (2017). *Psychodynamic Diagnostic Manual*, 2nd edition. New York and London: The Guilford Press.

Lorentzen, S., Bøgwald, K.-P., & Høglend, P. (2002). Change during and after Long-Term Analytic Group Psychotherapy. *International Journal Group Psychotherapy*, 52: 419–429.

Lorentzen, S., & Høglend, P. (2004). Predictors of Change during Long-Term Analytic Group Psychotherapy. *Psychotherapy and Psychosomatics*, 73: 25–35.

Lorentzen, S., Sexton, H., & Høglend, P. (2004). Therapeutic Alliance, Cohesion and Outcome in a Long-Term Analytic Group. *Nordic Journal of Psychiatry*, 58(1): 33–40.

Lorentzen, S., & Høglend, P. (2005). Predictors of Change during and after Long-Term Analytic Group Psychotherapy. *Journal of Clinical Psychology*, 61(12): 1541–1553.

Lorentzen, S. (2006). Contemporary Challenges for Research in Group Analysis. *Group Analysis*, 39(3): 321–340.

Lorentzen, S., & Høglend, P. (2008). Moderators of the Effects of Treatment Length in Long-Term Psychodynamic Group Psychotherapy. *Psychotherapy and Psychosomatics*, 77: 321–322.

Lorentzen, S., Ruud, T., Fjeldstad, A., & Høglend, P. (2013). Comparison of Short- and Long-Term Dynamic Group Psychotherapy: Randomised Clinical Trial. *British Journal of Psychiatry*, 203: 280–287.

Lorentzen, S. (2014). *Group Analytic Psychotherapy. Working with Affective, Anxiety and Personality Disorders*. London: Routledge.

Lorentzen, S., Fjeldstad, A., Ruud, T., & Høglend, P. (2015a). Comparing Short- and Long-Term Group Therapy: Seven-Year Follow-Up of a Randomized Clinical Trial. *Psychotherapy and Psychosomatics*, 84(5): 320–321.

Lorentzen, S., Fjeldstad, A., Ruud, T., Marble, A., Klungsøyr, O., Ulberg, R., & Høglend, P.A. (2015b). The Effectiveness of Short- and Long-Term Psychodynamic Group Psychotherapy on Self-Concept: Three Years Follow-Up of a Randomized Clinical Trial. *International Journal of Group Psychotherapy*, 65(4): 543–551.

Lorentzen, S., Ruud, T., Fjeldstad, A., & Høglend, P. (2015c). Personality Disorder Moderates Outcome in Short- and Long-Term Group Analytic Psychotherapy: A Randomized Clinical Trial. *British Journal of Clinical Psychology*, 54: 129–146.

Lorentzen, S., Strauss, B., & Altmann, U. (2018). Process-Outcome Relationships in Short- and Long-Term Psychodynamic Group Psychotherapy: Results from a Randomized Clinical Trial. *Group Dynamics: Theory, Research, and Practice*, 22(2): 93–107.

Lorentzen, S. (2022). *Focused Group Analytic Psychotherapy. An Integration of Clinical Experience and Research. An Integration of Clinical Experience and Research*. London and New York: Routledge.

Ogrodniczuk, J. (2006). Men, Women and Their Outcome in Psychotherapy. *Psychotherapy Research*, 16(4): 453–462.

OPD Task Force (Eds.). (2008). *Operationalized Psychodynamic Diagnosis OPD-2*. Göttingen, Germany: Hogrefe & Huber Publishers.

Pines, M. (Ed.). (1983). *The Evolution of Group Analysis*. London: Routledge and Kegan Paul.

Pines, M. (1994). The Group-as-a-Whole. In D. Brown, & L. Zinkin (Eds.) *The Psyche and the Social World* (pp. 47–59). London: Routledge.

Piper, W.E., McCallum, M., Joyce, A.S., Rosie, J.S., & Ogrodniczuk, J.S. (2001). Patient Personality and Time-Limited Group Psychotherapy for Complicated Grief. *International Journal of Group Psychotherapy*, 51(4): 525–552.

Schlapobersky, J.R. (2016). *From the Couch to the Circle. Group-Analytic Psychotherapy in Practice*. London and New York: Routledge.

Tasca, G.A., Ritchie, K., Conrad, G., Balfour, L., Gayton, J., Lybanon, V., & Bissada, H. (2006). Attachment Scales Predict Outcome in a Randomized Controlled Trial of Two Group Therapies for Binge Eating Disorder: An Aptitude by Treatment Interaction. *Psychotherapy Research*, 16: 106–121.

Yalom, I.D., & Leszcz, M. (2020). *The Theory and Practice of Group Psychotherapy*, 6th edition. New York: Basic Books.

# Part II
# Conceptual studies

# 7 Psychoanalysis and its distinct epistemology

*Erik Stänicke*

## Introduction[1]

Psychoanalysis and science have a long and intricate history. We may ask: What kind of science is psychoanalysis? Is psychoanalysis a scientific discipline or is it better labeled as art, a cultural movement, or even an ideology?[2] I will argue that psychoanalysis is a scientific discipline, but a distinctive one. I will present my view on philosophy of science and ask how psychoanalysis gathers and develops knowledge about the human mind. As psychoanalysts, we embrace knowledge – based on observations in the analytic situation – in an atypical manner. Our ideals are not – as for many other scientific enterprises – falsification on par with Karl Popper (1963). Scientific ideals are for most analysts not inspired by experimental design. Yet, some theories of ours are falsified – for example, Mahler´s theory of an autistic phase in the infant's development, and we also have examples of psychoanalytic theories having been tested in laboratories, such as Mark Solms' (2021) neuro-psychological testing of the Freudian hypothesis of dreams. My point is that these examples are exceptions. More typically, we analysts explore phenomena and develop theories about the mind and use them as 'thought-models'. I will present some characteristic features of thought-models and underline how these contrast to typical scientific ideals within academic psychology and medicine. This discrepant view on knowledge is a resource for us as analysts but is also controversial within academia. I will argue that psychoanalysis since Freud – indirectly with Klein and Winnicott, and more explicitly with Bion – is embedded in an epistemological position that can be traced back to the philosopher Immanuel Kant. Inspired by Kant's (1781) epistemological position of 'critical realism' or, more precisely stated, a modern reading of 'transcendental idealism', I highlight how main traditions within psychoanalysis view knowledge.

In this chapter, I will have two lines of thoughts on the question of psychoanalysis as science: First, I will argue that within psychoanalysis the status of theories is atypical, if I am correct, they are atypical especially if we compare the status of theories in other academic disciplines. Thus, I aim at

DOI: 10.4324/9781032651934-10

describing some characteristics of our take on theories. Second, I will argue that psychoanalysis has a specific epistemology which partly can shed light on the status of our theories.

## Psychoanalytic thought-models

Compared to mainstream academic psychology, psychoanalytic theories are characterized by atypical attributes (Stänicke & Lindstad 2020, 2021). Usually, theories in psychology are seen as kinds of models with a hypothetical status. Typically, psychological research consists in statistical probability testing of hypotheses. Thus, a psychological theory usually has status as being a more or less probable description or explanation of a phenomenon. For example, there exists research of how personality assessment predicts for different activities, such as success in work. Even in psychotherapy research, we find this kind of studies, for example, testing if a specific pathology theory in cognitive therapy has evidence or not. This is often not the case with psychoanalytic theories. We handle analytic theories – whether it is the Oedipus complex, projective identification, defense mechanisms, or the notion of unconscious phantasies – more as, what I will label as, 'thought-models'. These thought-models are seldomly tested and, even more rarely, falsified and rejected. It is as if we analysts collect them, some would say that we even hoard them. We apply theories more as regulative principles that may be relevant for our clinical practice, even when aspects or relations they refer to are not always manifested (ibid.). The advantage with thought-models is that they provide us with a rich resource of notions, models, and theories that we can make use of if they match our observation, thus helping us to meet patients as openly and neutrally as possible. More on this later.

Christopher Bollas (1989) has, in my opinion, described our attitudes toward psychoanalytic theories aptly. He writes that psychoanalytic theories may be illustrated – all the way back to Freud's theories on infantile sexuality, Oedipus complex, primary process thinking to modern object relation theory, or even modern mentalization theory – as being placed in a periodical system. In this periodical table, we have psychoanalytic concepts, notions, models, and theories standing side by side. Examples besides the ones already mentioned are alpha function, bi-logic, potential space, attachment, narcissistic needs, drive-affects, and death work – just to name some. All these thought-models have been developed by analysts aiming at describing their observations as truthfully as possible.

## Three features of psychoanalytic thought-models

I have claimed that psychoanalytic theories best can be understood as thought-models, instead of as probabilistic ones. From this claim, I want to promote three features of thought-models which I hope will make my claim more comprehensible and recognizable. First, I will argue that our thought-models, say of Oedipal complex, are about relations between causal dispositions in persons. Together with my colleague Tobias Lindstad (2020, 2021), I worked on integrating the idea of psychoanalytic thought-models with a dispositional account of causality as presented by Mumford and Anjum (2011). In this chapter, I will only illustrate shortly what a dispositional account of causality implies: The Oedipus complex refers to potential causal dispositions in a person. For example, a patient who report repetitive problems with social situations consisting of more than one other person, at the same time, being disturbed and anxious by the analyst's independent thinking – both cases referring to a triangulated situation – may direct our clinical thinking toward the model of Oedipus complex and transference. These thought-models sensitize us in our listening perspective for jealousy and loneliness (Britton 1989), and more specifically, for an understanding that the patient may be disposed for feeling neglected by the analyst. Hence, the thought-models in this case may aid the analyst to formulate interpretations. The properties and relations accounted for in a model – say the Oedipal complex – are not necessarily manifested in every context, but they can emerge in a specific analytic situation. Thus, even if a theory is not regularly observed, it may be shown to be relevant for understanding some unique patients.

Second, thought-models are characterized by being regulative principles, sometimes idealized principles, contrary to a constitutive one. A constitutive principle refers to rules or laws, that applies in every situation. Psychoanalytic models are not of that stature. Rather, our models are regulative, they refer to dispositions that may become manifest in some contexts and with some patients, but not every time. An example is our concept of analytic neutrality. As Bjørn Killingmo (1997) writes in a seminal article on abstinence, it does not imply that analysts should behave according to an ideal of being neutral in every situation, nor does it imply being cold and inhuman. Contrary, abstinence is best understood as a regulative principle for understanding the curative action of psychoanalysis that aid the analyst in recognizing when a response or intervention is an exception from usual practice. For example, as analyst we listen for the patient's subtext and transference, and thus are cautious of answering questions on face value. However, that does not mean that we never can or even should answer questions on face value. In some contexts, it is the only right thing to do, but without rejecting the concept of neutrality. Not at all, neutrality aids us in thinking it through when to do what, so we do not only respond on impulse but try to understand clinical transactions and communications in light of the unconscious.

Third, thought-models are elastic – as Sandler (1983) has argued. Psychoanalytic theories and concepts are elastic in the sense that they are not operationalized in a limited way. The analyst uses theories as models to reflect on clinical matters and thus does not search for a perfect fit between a theory and a phenomenon. The aim for the analyst is not to 'prove' to himself that a theory confirms a phenomenon, but rather let the theory aid us into thinking and finding interpretations that are helpful for the patient. Even if this elasticity violates the scientific ideal of precision, I think that analysts still strive for precision, but will not let it stand in the way of vital clinical thinking and facilitation of the analytic process.

I want to make a qualification on thought-models. One objection may be that there exists psychoanalytic research that do not fit with the idea of thought-models. And, as I mentioned in the Introduction, there are exceptions. For example, the research of Mark Solms on the brain with psychoanalytic models or the studies of Peter Fonagy on attachment, mentalization, and epistemic trust take place more along regular academic ideals. I am not aiming at reflecting on their research, it is well versed by their own doing. My argument in this chapter is more about how we as clinical analysts develop, handle, and think about our theories and knowledge.

## Thought-models embedded in a Kantian epistemology

My claim that psychoanalytic theories do not aim for the same scientific ideals as mainstream research within academic psychology and psychiatry must be further elaborated. What does the claim of thought-models imply? And, in what overarching epistemology is psychoanalysis embedded? At first glance, it can seem unscientific to state that theories are not falsifiable, but hoarded in a periodical system, that they are not operationalized, but are kept elastic. With Karl Popper (1963) such a claim would underscore psychoanalysis as pseudo-scientific. However, I do not think that these features throw us out from the good company of science. Rather, psychoanalysis as a scientific enterprise has a specific epistemological position. In my opinion, this specific position also makes further sense to the idea of thought-models.

As mentioned in the beginning, there is a long debate about the scientific status of psychoanalysis. However, the underlying question of the epistemological position of psychoanalysis is not much debated although there have been some intense debates about psychoanalysis being a science conforming to ideals from positivism or social-constructionism (Hoffman 1991). Another contender in the debate, especially well argued by Charles Hanly (1995, 1999, 2009, 2020), has been 'critical realism'. In the overall sense, I agree with Hanly that psychoanalysis can best be understood within critical realism, but I will argue that it can be even better understood within the philosopher Immanuel Kant's (1781) position of transcendental idealism.

I will in the following qualify in what way psychoanalysis is embedded in a Kantian epistemology, as at face value, there is a large discrepancy between Kant and Freud (see also Stänicke et al. 2020). But before we investigate their differences, I will make you attentive to traits in Freud's thinking that illustrate how influenced he seems of a Kantian worldview. First, Freud shared Kant's strong confidence in rationality. One of Freud's (1933) most notorious citations is: 'Our best hope for the future is that intellect – the scientific spirit, reason – may in the process of time establish a dictatorship in the mental life of man' (p. 171). This statement demonstrates Freud's unwavering belief in rationality – probably never claimed as strongly as with Kant before him. Second, Freud argues that we cannot grasp truth directly, but only approach it through our representations of the world and ourselves. In a line from 1900, Freud almost paraphrases Kant:

> The unconscious is the true psychical reality; in its innermost nature it is as much unknown to us as the reality of the external world, and it is as incompletely presented by the data of consciousness as is the external world by the communications of our sense organs.
>
> (p. 613)

Freud's Kantian take on rationality and the epistemological view that the world is not given to us seems to me to have retained its strong position in psychoanalysis after Freud, while it has probably faded in other academic disciplines. As I will argue, this matter may partly explain the misunderstandings and controversies we see between academic psychology and psychoanalysis.

Thus, there are some, very important, parallels between Freud and Kant, yet there are also huge differences. Even if Freud agrees with Kant that the subject is not transparent to himself, a difference is that for Kant this lack of transparency is epistemological but for Freud it is psychological. Thus, what for Kant is a lack in epistemological transparency – in what the subject can know about the world – is also a universal lack, but for Freud the lack of transparency is mostly dynamic and can even be improved by analysis. There are of course many other differences between the two thinkers, yet, in this context, their different understanding of the subject's lack is fundamental.

Notwithstanding their differences, there are good reasons to read Freud as being highly influenced and inspired by Kant's rationalism in general and epistemological position specifically. Alfred Tauber (2009, 2010) has argued convincingly that Freud aimed at integrating a humanistic psychological project with a scientific enterprise on par with medicine. This is a way of reading Freud's project as in one way being both social-constructionistic and positivistic. Tauber argues that this strain in Freud could have been more clear for later generations if he had clarified that he was inspired by his contemporary neo-Kantian Zeitgeist.

My proposition is that Freud's epistemological position as a Kantian one can be further clarified if we read Kant anew. One challenge with reading Kant today is that there are so many ways of interpreting his work. I will make use of one of today's most influential and authoritative Kant readers,

Henry Allison (2004), in order to present an epistemological position that I aim at making recognizable for many analysts and that more specifically can make sense of our way of using theories. But before I go into the complicated matter, let me summarize the overall epistemological project that Kant established.

Kant was trained as a rationalist that holds the view that any knowledge of significance – knowledge that are universally true – can only be sourced in the inner forms of rationality by reflexive thinking. However, when he read David Hume's presentation of empiricism he aimed at bridging this with his rationalistic viewpoint. Empiricism holds that all universal truths can only be reached through our senses. By systemizing our observations and describing them as accurately as possible, we can gradually develop true knowledge about ourselves and the world. Roughly stated, rationalism at its end-point leads us to idealism, while empiricism leads into naïve realism. Hence, while rationalism advices us to explore our representations and way of thinking self-critically in order to attain knowledge, empiricism advices us systematically to observe, describe, and be critical about any biases we can have in this endeavor.

Kant's philosophical achievement was to integrate these two epistemological positions by claiming that thinking about objects should lead us to observe the world, while at the same time we should also think about our knowledge in order to grasp how rationality constitutes reality. There are a lot of philosophical technicalities that does not need to worry us in this context. The crucial point now is that Kant explores the conditions for our observations and thinking about the world. The conditions are that no object can exist in our mind without it being structured by time and space, and that objects can causally influence each other, just to name some of them. Kant's famous Copernican revolution consists of revealing that we as rational beings form, in the sense constitute, the world we gain knowledge about, instead of the naïve understanding of us humans getting knowledge about objects in the world that impinge our senses.

Summarized, a Kantian epistemology provides an argument for being an empirical realist – as researchers or, in our case, as analysts – but at the same time highlighting, in line with rationalism, that our observation of ourselves and the world always are in discourse with concepts. Our knowledge is always conveyed through our representations, and thus never directly registered through our senses. This point of not having direct access to knowledge about ourselves or the world, but only mediated by representations, is what Kant wanted to stress with his concept of 'things-in-themselves' not being known by us. Henry Allison (2004), the well-known Kantian expert, argues that things-in-themselves must be understood in light of, what he calls, a 'two-aspect' view. Let me cite Allison to make his argument clear: 'In other words, the claim is not that *things* transcending the condition of human cognition cannot exist, but merely that such things cannot count as objects for us' (ibid., p. 12). He then argues that such a reading provides 'a doctrine of epistemological modesty' (ibid., p. xvi). The modesty refers to us humans as finite observers and thinkers that can never achieve a 'God's-eye view' of things.

You may ask, who claim to have a 'God's-eye view' in science, or in our case, as analysts. According to Kant transcendental realists do, which he connects to both rationalists and empiricists. The point Kant wants to make is that the possibility of providing new knowledge requires both concepts, as in representations, and sensible intuition, as in observations (Allison 2004).

### Epistemology in object relation theory

Having made the claim that Freud is invested in this Kantian epistemology, I will further argue that later object relational theory, as developed by Klein, Winnicott, and Bion, implicitly applied the same epistemology without stating it. Bion is the exception, because he is quite explicitly influenced by Kant's epistemology, as well as Kant's framework and theories (see also Stänicke et al. 2020).

As is well-known, Melanie Klein (1952) argues that the infant develops from an immature position – which she calls the schizoid-paranoid position – to a more mature depressive position. This development consists of several things, but in our context, it is of significance that the gradual development of the ego consists of an increased 'comprehension of the world': 'Accordingly, the picture of his (the infant's) parents, which was at first distorted into idealized and terrifying figures, comes gradually nearer to reality' (Klein 1952, p. 74). The crucial point here is the explicit statement of 'gradually nearer to reality', which implies that reality is never grasped completely or once and for all, but is something we struggle to perceive and comprehend.

Winnicott has another take on the matter, but he also only states his epistemology indirectly as Klein did. His developmental theory is different from Klein's in stressing the infant's need of good-enough mothering in establishing an intermediate area in the development from pleasure to reality principle (Winnicott 1953). Let me quote Winnicott's famous line: 'The baby creates the object, but the object was there waiting to be created and to become a cathected object' (1971, p. 89). This statement expresses quite clearly Winnicott's understanding of how our possibility to establish knowledge happens through concurrent concepts and observations, as I argued with Kant.

With Bion we find an explicit reference to Kant. He refers to Kant's concept of 'thing-in-itself' as beta-elements (Bion 1962), later referring to O as 'a thing-in-itself and unknowable' (1965, pp. 12–13). Kant seems to have been important for Bion's development of a theory of thinking. He pictures the infant with inborn pre-conceptions or disposition to experience significant parts of reality. His main example is how the infant has an expectation of the breast, as a kind of a priori knowledge – an 'empty thought' that exists before experience, but that can be actualized into a conception of the breast if the infant has an appropriate experience. Here we can see the concurrent theory of Kant. The concurrent need of perception and concept that I talked about earlier, in order to make experience and knowledge, is fully taken in use by Bion.

## Critical realism and transcendental idealism

Kant's epistemology – which he quirkily named 'transcendental idealism' – suits psychoanalysis providing a basis for us to be realists, but in a modest way since it also encourages us to critically examine our representations of reality. This is a position that has affinity with Roy Bhaskar's epistemological position of critical realism (see Benton & Craib 2010). In psychoanalysis, critical realism has been elegantly worked out by Charles Hanly (1995, 1999; Hanly & Hanly 2001, 2020). Hanly (1995) writes, 'we depend on ideas to understand, ideas also have the potential to distort' (p. 906). Hence, critical realism is all about being suspicious about being wrong or, as we understand it in psychoanalysis, self-deceptive ideas. Thus, critical realism seems to be a contender for psychoanalytic epistemology, however, there are some problems with this position that Kant warned us about.

The problem with critical realism is that it aims to state facts about reality. Kant warns about the pitfalls with what he calls transcendental realism – which critical realism is – in that it implies that even if reality is transcendent to our representation of it, it can be grasped and registered. I will argue that – educated by Kant, Freud, and also Bion – we should be modest about our truth claims. Having experience with the unconscious, we know that we can never be totally transparent in our truth claims; there will always be desires and destructive motives in our contact with reality. Or to allude to Kant, our grasp of reality can never be with the thing-in-itself, it is always mediated through our human perspective. With Allison's words (2004), we can never get a God-eye-view on the world or ourselves. What Kant reminds us of is the limit of our knowledge. This way of understanding knowledge production was part of Freud's academic training in a central Europe that was invested in neo-Kantian thinking.

## Conclusion

Our slowly developed psychoanalytic theories have distinct features, as I have argued in this chapter, of being models for thought rather than predictions that can be verified or falsified. A trait of psychoanalytic knowledge is that we do not discard theories, but instead harbor them for a time where we meet a patient that seems to struggle with a kind of concern that can be of need of a specific model. For example, the Freudian version of Oedipus complex is not that frequently relevant for a typical patient of today.

Yet, suddenly there comes a time where it is exactly what is needed. We can then see the model as a representation of reality – in line with Kant's epistemology – that can be of use with a specific patient in a given session. However, we know that today's session can only – to paraphrase Andre Green – be understood tomorrow. Thus, an interpretation of Oedipus complex in a Monday session may be understood as wrong in a Tuesday session. The patient had a dream in between the two sessions that invites us to think along different models and theories. Hence, our psychoanalytic knowledge is on par with a Kantian epistemology – transcendental idealism – and our theories are like thought-models that more or less represent a given reality but are never things-in-themselves. Hence, psychoanalysis seems deeply indebted to Kant's modest epistemology.

## Notes

1  A preliminary version of this chapter was originally presented at the EPF conference 2022 in Vienna and that presentation is published in EPF Bulletin. This chapter is an integration of thinking published in three separate papers (Stänicke et al. 2020; Stänicke & Lindstad 2020, 2021).
2  For further reflections on these questions, see Marianne Leuzinger-Bohleber's (2023) enlightening discussion.

## References

Allison, H.E. (2004). *Kant's Transcendental Idealism: An Interpretation and Defense.* New Haven, CT: Yale University Press.
Benton, T. & Craib, I. (2010). *Philosophy of Social Science: The Philosophical Foundations of Social Thought.* New York: Palgrave Macmillan.
Bion, W.R. (1962). *Learning from Experience.* London: Karnac, 1984.
Bion, W.R. (1965). Transformations. In Seven Servants. New York: Jason Aronson, 1977.
Bollas, C. (1989). *Forces of Destiny: Psychoanalysis and Human Idiom.* Abingdon: Routledge.
Britton, R. (1989). The Missing Link: Parental Sexuality in the Oedipus Complex. In J. Steiner (ed.) *The Oedipus Complex Today: Clinical Implications.* London: Karnac.
Freud, S. (1900). The Interpretation of Dreams. SE 5:509–621.
Freud, S. (1933). New Introduction Lectures on Psycho-Analysis. SE 22:1–182.
Hanly, C. (1995). On Fact and Ideas in Psychoanalysis. International Journal of Psychoanalysis **76**:901–908.
Hanly, C. (1999). On Subjectivity and Objectivity in Psychoanalysis. International Journal of Psychoanalysis **47**:427–444.
Hanly, C. & Hanly, M.A. (2001). Critical Realism: Distinguishing the Psychological Subjectivity of the Analyst from Epistemological Subjectivism. International Journal of Psychoanalysis **49**:515–532.
Hanly, C. (2009). On Truth and Clinical Psychoanalysis. International Journal of Psychoanalysis **90**: 363–373.
Hanly, C. (2020). Psychoanalytic Epistemology: Kant and Freud. *Psychoanalytic Quarterly* **89**(2): 305–337.

Hoffman, I.Z. (1991). Discussion: Toward a Social-Constructivist view of the Psychoanalytic Situation. *Psychoanalytic Dialogues* **1**:74–105.

Kant, I. (1781). *Critique of Pure Reason*. Cambridge: Cambridge University Press, 1997.

Killingmo, B. (1997). The So-called Rule of Abstinence Revisited. Scandinavian Psychoanalytic Review **20**:144–159.

Klein, M. (1952). Some Theoretical Conclusions Regarding the Emotional Life of the Infant. In M. Klein (ed.) *The Writings of Melanie Klein, III*. London: Hogarth Press, 1975, pp. 61–92.

Leuzinger-Bohleber, M. (2023). Introduction: On the Dark Side: Chronic Depression and Trauma – Signatures of Our Time? Some Societal, Conceptual and Methodological Considerations. In M. Leuzinger-Bohleber, G. Ambresin, T. Fischmann & M. Solms (ed.) On the Dark Side of Chronic Depression: Psychoanalytic, Social-cultural and Research Approaches. Oxon: Routledge, pp. 1–30.

Mumford, S. & Anjum, R.L. (2011). Getting Causes from Powers. Oxford Academic.

Popper, K.R. (1963). *Conjectures and Refutations*. London: Routledge.

Solms, M. (2021). Hidden Spring: A Journey to the Source of Consciousness. London: Profile Books.

Sandler, J. (1983). Reflections on Some Relations between Psychoanalytic Concepts and Psychoanalytic Practice. International Journal of Psychoanalysis **64**:35–45.

Stänicke, E. & Lindstad, T. (2020). The Pragmatic Status of Psychoanalytic Theory: A Plea for Thought Models. In T. Lindstad, E. Stänicke & J. Valsiner (Red.) Respect for Thought: Jan Smedslund's Legacy for Psychology. Cham: Springer, pp. 377–400.

Stänicke, E. & Lindstad, T. (2021). The Catalytic Powers of Psychoanalytic Thought Models. In B. Wagoner, B.A. Christensen & C. Demuth (Red.) Culture as Process: A Tribute to Jaan Valsiner. Cham: Springer, pp. 419–429.

Stänicke, E., Zachrisson, A. & Vetlesen, A.J. (2020). The Epistemological Stance of Psychoanalysis: Revisiting the Kantian Legacy. *The Psychoanalytic Quarterly* **89**(2): 281–304.

Tauber, A.I. (2009). Freud's Dreams of Reason: The Kantian Structure of Psychoanalysis. *History of the Human Sciences* **22**:1–29.

Tauber, A.I. (2010). *Freud: The Reluctant Philosopher*. Princeton, NJ: Princeton University Press.

Winnicott, D.W. (1953). Transitional Objects and Transitional Phenomena. In D. Winnicott (ed.) *Playing and Reality*. London and New York: Routledge, 1971, pp. 1–25.

Winnicott, D.W. (1971). The Use of an Object and Relating through Identifications. In D. Winnicott (ed.) *Playing and Reality*. London and New York: Routledge, pp. 86–94.

# 8 Self-agency and self-reflection – building blocks for a dual self theory

*Werner Bohleber*

## Preliminary remarks

Anthropologically, an essential characteristic of man is his self-reflexivity. The singularity of self-reflection lies in the fact that the individual self can relate to itself dialogically. Simultaneously, it is able to place itself above itself and, through this, again is able to relate to this self-relation. In this way, the self is in a constant relationship to itself. The motor for the self-reflexive processes is the agency of the self. Thus, a self occurs that has two aspects, one in which it appears as a mental actor and one in which it becomes an object of observation for itself.

To attain self-knowledge is a goal of psychoanalytic treatment. In psychoanalysis, this has been discussed since the 1950s by the concept of insight. The fact that self-reflection with its mental functions forms the more comprehensive framework, which makes insight first possible, remained largely out of consideration. One reason for this was the fact that the psychoanalytic structural theory could not adequately address the inner capacity of the self for reflection.

These brief preliminary remarks outline the structure of my contribution. I will begin with some comments on the concept of the self in psychoanalysis, and then go further and discuss theories which try to conceptualize its inner dialogical capacity. Building on this, I will present some basic features of the dual structure of the self. In a final section, I want to outline how the concept of a dual self can provide a better understanding of the psychic processes of insight.

## The concept of the self in psychoanalysis

The psychoanalytic literature on the concept of the self manifests considerable confusion, which does not always make it easy to find one's way through the various conceptions. Freud used the concept of the ego both for the whole person and for a psychic substructure. He never cleared up this ambiguity, but always maintained the inner tension of his concept of the ego (Laplanche & Pontalis 1988). His interest was in the metapsychological

DOI: 10.4324/9781032651934-11

structural ego, condemning the holistic self of experience to a shadowy existence. It only appeared when Freud personified the psychic agencies and spoke, for example, of the "poor ego". As result the subjective phenomenological self no longer had a place in theory, and with it any attempt to adequately conceptualize the self-reflection which is so central to the psychoanalytic cure.

It was then Heinz Hartmann (1950) who separated the two aspects of the Freudian ego and introduced the concept of the self. He tried to solve the conceptual problems that this separation caused for the structural model by excluding the structural properties of the self and integrating it into the structure of the ego, now narrowing the self down to the experiential concept of self-representation. To speak of self-representation then became common in psychoanalysis to conceptualize the psychic content of the self. The problems arising from this solution determined the psychoanalytic discussion for decades, until – beginning with Heinz Kohut – conceptions of the self emerged that left the structural model behind. I cannot elaborate on this here, but I would like to point out that in the whole discussion an essential characteristic of the human self was only mentioned in passing or not at all, namely its *reflexive structure,* which makes it first possible for human beings to think about themselves. Instead, we find terms like "self-observation", "introspection", "self-knowledge", and "insight". But which mental functions are exactly meant by these terms remains largely an open question. It is therefore no coincidence that in most treatment theories the concept of self-reflection hardly occurs. Although Richard Sterba (1934) and Robert Waelder (1934) took up the philosophical concept of self-reflection in the 1930s and tried to integrate it in psychoanalytic theory, this anthropological horizon was lost again. Greenson (1967), for example, speaks only of a split in ego functions between a rational, observing, analyzing ego and an experiencing, subjective, irrational ego .

In order to adequately grasp self-reflection and self-knowledge, we need a theory that can describe the reflexive structure of the self. In the search for it, we come across the self-theories of William James and George Herbert Mead.

### The dual structure of the self

In his famous work "The Principles of Psychology" (1892/1902) William James writes that every psychology must start from the fundamental fact that "the consciousness of Self involves a stream of thought" (1892, 215), in which thoughts, feelings, and mental states emerge and disappear again according to their own laws. The whole self has a dual structure. Partly it is the knower, partly the known, partly subject, partly object. James calls one part of the self the "I" and the other the "Me". But both parts do not fall apart. They are one and yet differentiated (1892, 176). The "I" is the "thinker", it isn't an entity, but a thought, "at each moment different from that of the last moment, but appropriative of the latter". It can only be aware of itself in the *act of* thought. It is more or less a pure awareness. If the "I" tries to think about itself concretely, it can only do it with the help of the "Me"-aspect. The "Me", on the other hand, is the empirical self, an aggregate of its states of consciousness, its psychic properties, and dispositions. If the self as an "I" it can take itself as an object and as a "me" it is perceiving itself as an Other. Through this both parts of the self can have a dialogue with each other based on a social communication process, which the child has introjected in its socialization.

George Herbert Mead explains this fact psychologically. For him, too, the self is formed[1] by the "I" and the "Me", they are both phases of the self. The "Me" arises from innumerable internalization and identification processes. The child internalizes social role expectations. Mead speaks here of the "generalized other", referring to the respective social rules of behavior, roles, norms, and values. The "I" is the "principle of action and impulse" (Mead 1934, 27). In taking itself as an object, the "I" must adopt the perspective of social others vis-à-vis itself, for it can only know itself on the basis of given roles and socially preformed expectations. But since it adopts them in a most individual way, it can decide for itself whether and how to make something its own. This provides it with innovative leeway (Tugendhat 1979, 279).

While for James the "I" was ultimately the dynamic activity of the self and its pure awareness, Mead goes beyond this and endows the "I" with a pre-reflexive spontaneity and creativity, but also with libidinal impulses, which, however, he understands more generally as driving activity and not only as libido and aggression. Such a theory of the self, based on James and Mead, was revolutionary for the time of the 1920s in psychology and social sciences.

At the same time as Mead, representatives of Philosophical Anthropology in Germany developed ideas and concepts that have a striking similarity to James' and Mead's conceptions of the self. Above all, the contributions of Helmuth Plessner deserved to be mentioned here. Plessner conceptualizes the dual structure of the self as the "eccentric positionality" of man, which enables him to see himself from the outside. The self, therefore, has two poles, an "I" as the subject pole, a "pure I" that cannot be objectified, and an experiential representational "me" that is realized in social roles (1928, 364). Plessner conceptualizes the "pure" nonobjectifiable "I" more substantially than James and Mead. It enables humans to engage in ever new acts of reflection on themselves. However, these reflections can never be able to come to an end, which is why personal individuality ultimately remains incomprehensible even to its own "I" (an *individuum ineffabile*) (1961, 201). Its nonobjectifiable character also makes the "I" socially "untouchable" and creates for it a "reservoir of privacy" from social demands. We find similar ideas of the self in psychoanalysis in Winnicott and Modell. I will come back to it. Plessner had to emigrate during the Nazi era, so that his work was only gradually being received after the Second World War.

How have psychoanalysts taken up these basic ideas of a dual self-structure and conceived them psychoanalytically? In the recent years, Peter Fonagy and his research group (2002) have taken up William James' "I" and "Me" for their developmental theory of mentalization. From earlier years, the most important contributions to be mentioned are those of Erik Erikson, Donald Winnicott, Arnold Modell, and Jacques Lacan. The focus of my own thinking on the theory of the dual self is on the study of self-reflection. I will therefore limit myself in the following to a discussion of the self-theories of Erikson, Winnicott, and Modell.

## Erik Erikson's dual conception of identity

Erikson had studied art before coming into contact with psychoanalysis (Friedman 1999). Art had awakened his particular interest in how the inner emotional world finds shape and form in outer reality. He developed a "configurational approach" in which he always sought to think the inner world together with the outer reality. The external world did not have a restrictive or endangering character for him as it did for Anna Freud, but he was interested in the convergences, how the outside meets the inside, how the two fit together and produce specific psychosocial configurations. After migrating to the United States, Erikson came into contact with the psychology of William James and George Herbert Mead. Their conceptions of "I" and "Me" gave him new impulses for the development of his concept of identity. Erikson (1968) distinguishes an "I-aspect" from a "Self-aspect" in identity formation. The I is a "central and partly unconscious organizing agent". Its task is to reflect the representations and identifications of the self that have been formed through social realization and to bring them into attunement with one another. If the integration of self-images succeeds, it finally culminates in a sense of identity. The sense of identity becomes the supreme principle, evaluating and regulating the dynamic interaction of the organizing I with the respective real self-realizations. Therefore, a sense of identity is not a state, but as an organ of regulation it is involved in a reflexive process between I and Me.

Erikson always wanted to reconcile his conception of the psyche with Freud's structural theory. He separated the Freudian ego into two parts (1968). The "I" is the conscious organ capable of reflection, while the ego as the "Me"-aspect operates unconsciously, organizing perceptions, feelings, impulses, and memories and ensuring the continuity of our existence. But this attempt didn't work. The Freudian ego cannot replace the conscious I as a central instance capable of reflection. Erikson emphasizes that psychoanalysis has denied this organ of self-consciousness and self-reflection that makes self-analysis possible. For him (1970), this "I" has an "autonomy" and independence (Eigenständigkeit) that enables it to transcend its roles and the place it has taken in society. In an identity crisis, it is able to overcome inner and outer developmental limitations and to realign its identity.

## Donald Winnicott's theory of the self

Winnicott appreciated Erikson's work. Similarities are obvious in some of their concepts, such as the importance of the early mother relationship for the formation of the self and for the development of basic trust. In Erikson, identity formation has a dual aspect of self-creation and recognition (actualization) by the social environment, while Winnicott understands this dual aspect quite similarly as a paradox of creating and being found (1965, 250). Explicitly, Winnicott compared Erikson's "in-between" position of identity that mediates the outside with the inside to his conception of intermediary space (1971, 59). Winnicott's "true self" has similarities to Erikson's "I" and his "false self" embodies portions of the psychosocial self.

Jan Abram emphasizes that Winnicott's work can rightly be considered a theory of the self (2007, 5ff). While much of his work has been widely received, the same cannot be said of his theory of the self. For Winnicott, it is central to the infant's sense of self that the mother adapts sufficiently well and contingently to her infant and his needs. Contingent provision paves the way in the infant for an omnipotent illusion that he himself created the object. It is a first experience of agency, reinforced by the spontaneous gestures in which he can discover his own self and successively acquire the ability to be alone. In the spontaneous gesture, the true self comes into action. The true self is not a purely psychic entity, but it is also fed by the totality of sensorimotor aliveness (1965, 194). Progressive cognitive development gradually enables the young child to recognize the illusory element in his experience of omnipotence and to transfer it to play and fantasy (1960/1965, 146). For further development, the adaptation of the true self to social situations is required. To adequately capture the difficulties of this process, Winnicott introduces a duality of the self and differentiates between a true and a false self.

The false self represents for him that part of the self which, turned outward, is in connection with the world. It is important to understand that the false self isn't only negative but that it also plays a positive function. Through its "compliance", it can adapt and seek conditions "which will make it possible for the true self to come into its own" and to preserve its creativity and spontaneity through participation in cultural experience (1960/1965, 143). The true self, in turn, has the function of challenging the social realizations of the false self, especially when it, instead of seeking genuine compromise, tends toward conformity (compliance). In this case, when the degree of split between them is pathologically high, we find a compliant false self – rather than an adaptive false self – that hides the true self in such a way that it no longer has access to it. When the degree of split is low and healthy, both remain in contact with each other.

Yet the true self has still one additional aspect for Winnicott. It is a personal core of the self which is "an incommunicado element". Despite all communication with the world, "each individual is an isolate, permanently non-communicating, permanently unknown, in fact unfound" (ibid., 187). This "non-communicating central self" is silent to the outside world, but it has a kind of communication with itself that is "like music of the spheres, absolutely personal. It belongs to being alive" (ibid., 102). What Winnicott has in mind here, but does not reflect further, is in my opinion the basic affective atmosphere of the core self, which has been generated by the early interactions with the primary object. If we listen quietly into ourselves, we can perceive it in a rudimentary way. But in such an absolutely personal inner communication, as Winnicott is conceiving it, the self is again doubled into an "I"-aspect and a "Me"-aspect.

## Arnold Modell's theory of the self

Arnold Modell (1993, 2008) bases his conception of the self on James, Winnicott, and on the neurobiologist Gerald Edelman. For Modell, the self is an agent that is superior to all other mental structures. The human subject is embodied and its self must be grounded in psychobiology for otherwise we cannot adequately conceptualize coherence and continuity of self-experience. The self is dependent on social recognition, but yet not entirely, for a part of it can become autonomous and free itself from dependence on social recognition. Modell calls this aspect of the self that can have internal autonomy "private self", referring to Winnicott's "true self" and to James's "spiritual self". The private self can experience itself when it is in a state of "non-being-in-relation". Then it can experience itself as its very own. The strength of the private self is derived not only from its involvement in social structures, but essentially also from the inner contact with its basic affective core, which Modell anchors not only in relational experiences of early childhood, but also in the biological core self described by neuroscience. This gives the self with a firm ground for its capacity for autonomy, which protects it from becoming wholly dependent on social recognition. The psychobiological matrix provides the self with a paradoxical structure. On the one hand, it has a sense of deeply anchored continuity, and on the other hand it can be an ever-changing momentary consciousness at the same time. This paradox enables the self to keep its distance from the inputs of the immediate present and thus be able "to be free of the 'tyranny' of ongoing events in real time" (Modell 1993, 71).

## Interim summary

Let us summarize how these three theories conceptualize the dual self-aspects "I" and "Me" and their interaction. Erikson has described the dual process structure of the self in the most sophisticated way. The I as a reflective central agency organizes the self-representations for the formation of an identity. In Winnicott, the true self functions as the guardian of a social living self that strives to lead a meaningful authentic existence.

The structural parallelism of the true and false self with the "I" and "Me" -aspects is obvious. Modell emphasizes the psychobiological matrix that provides continuity and coherence to the self. Winnicott's concept of the non-communicating central self which "belongs to being alive" tries to conceptualize something similar. Modell's "private self" has similarities to Winnicott's "true self", but it also has features of Erikson's "I", which, through its inner autonomy and reflexive capacity, allows the empirical "Me" a certain freedom to change.

Although they seek to capture the self differently, all three theories agree on one point: They bring back into theory the aspect of personal whole-ness and individuality that Freud had not conceptually explored. They are able to describe the unresolvable tension that manifests itself in every individual existence between being a subject and its social representational realization.

The duality of the self is the basis for the processes of self-reflection, but all three theories do not explore this point further. I would like to consider some of these processes in more detail.

### The self as mental agent and self-reflection[2]

As psychoanalysts we are used to analyzing mental events post factum. Our main subject is the world of the representational self or, in other words, the world of mentalized experience. Hardly once we are concerned with the now-moment of experience itself. The situation has already changed slightly, if we think of the concept of intersubjective encounter or of Daniel Stern's "now-moments" (2004). My special interest is focused on the fact, that in the now-moment, there is a moment of pure experience, which with its quality as an "event" (similar to the Greek kairos) is standing transverse to the course of chronological time. Experience has an immediate occur-rence, but it can only be made comprehensible to us in its mediated form as mental representation. Nevertheless, we cannot avoid conceptualizing this moment of "pure" experience. James chose the concept of the I as "pure" initiative for this purpose. Mead defined the I as the "pre-reflective, spon-taneous, impulsive and creative dimensions of human agency" (cited in Dews 1995, 505). In the psychoanalytic literature, it has become common to speak of this aspect of the self as its "agency". However, the term is not clearly defined.

In our effort to conceptualize the agency aspect of the self, the findings of recent studies in developmental psychology are of help. In the 1980s in-fant research gave new impulses to the study of the self. I summarize some of the findings relevant to us. Because the mother regularly regulates and satisfies the infant's states, configurations of expectations are established in the infant. By satisfying them, the mother makes sure that a feeling can arise in the infant that he or she can directly influence its own state and steer it in the desired direction. This creates in the infant a sense of being able to bring about the desired states itself as the agent (Sander 2008, 287). Winnicott had already described this state of affairs. For him, the contingent satisfaction of needs by the mother paves the way in the infant for an omnipotent illusion that he himself has created the object. These first experiences of agency are reinforced by "spontaneous gestures" made by the infant during periods of undisturbed attention in which a "primary endogenous activity" can unfold. Both the intersubjective and individual forms of self-state regulation are driven by many other developmental processes, leading to a coherent sense of the self-as-agent (Sander 2008, 287). Peter Fonagy and his research group (Fonagy et al. 2002) have shown that agency is a major developmental factor for the mental self. Through various stages, self-agency develops into the acquisition of a historical-causal concept of an autobiographical self.

In summary, a central finding from all this research is that the emergence of self-consciousness merges with the sense of one's own agency. Agency constitutes the vitality and transformative power of the self. It is, so to speak, the fuel for one's own thinking and action but also for self-reflection.

On the role that the agency of the self plays in the act of self-reflection, I can only make a few comments here from a phenomenological perspective. Self-reflection is always an act of self-externalization. When we take ourselves as object, the self with its agency rises out of the stream of consciousness and detaches itself from the representational world. However, this psychic process is not a detachment, but the self-as-agent remains connected to the representational self, it can only "transcend" it in order to be able to reflexively turn back on itself and its representational world. In this act of transcending, a particular sense of agency comes into action that gives the self a sense of momentary freedom despite all psychic determination (something similar Waelder sought to describe in 1934). The analytic concept of free association also borrows from this sense of freedom, which is made possible by reflexive distance.

### Self-reflection and the concept of insight in psychoanalytic treatment technique

The metacognitive ability to reflect on oneself has not yet been sufficiently studied in its importance for analytic work. Therefore, I would like to conclude by showing how a new understanding of the dual self with its phases of the I and the Me can contribute to the concept of insight.

Insight as a technical concept of treatment has been an issue in psychoanalysis since the 1950s. The debate about it were later replaced by the topic of the curative factors of the therapeutic relationship. Insight is always a reflection on oneself through which we gain a new or more differentiated view of ourselves. In insight the dual structure of the self is at work: Insight has the character of an event. In the self-reflective act, the new view of the mental situation in question that emerges through the interpretation shatters the previous mental equilibrium and thereby enables a mental re-structuring. It is a process that is set in motion and also controlled by the agentive self. The cognitive-affective content of the insight can only unfold afterwards and is descriptively grasped and psychologically integrated by the representational self.

In the literature, a distinction is usually made between emotional and descriptive insight. Jerome Richfield (1954) clarified this distinction with his concept of "ostensive insight", referring to Bertrand Russel's distinction between "knowledge by acquaintance" and "knowledge by description". He described an important condition that must be given for the psychic process of insight to be able to get underway at all. It consists in the fact that the current transference relationship must have an intense affective quality for the patient. If the analyst, in his interpretation, brings together the present experience with old patterns of experience of it, an immediately emerging new view becomes possible which restructures the cognitive-affective field. The condition for this is that the *act* of insight takes place suddenly and immediately and, as with a flash, illuminates the inner field and thereby opens a new view of oneself.

This psychic immediacy has been shown to be an essential criterion for insight and conviction. James Strachey (1934) already emphasized the importance of intense affective experience and immediacy as an essential moment of action in a mutative interpretation. Warren Poland has further clarified the meaning of immediacy. He writes:

> Addressing the immediacy of the psychic moment gives an interpretation its impact, even when it is the historical past that is under discussion. A person's mind is entire. Examination of any part, past or present, content or process, is alive in the experience of the immediate moment if it rings true as an authentic part of discovery and working through.
>
> (1988, 352)

Only this "analytic immediacy" makes meanings really meaningful for the patient and transforms analytic facts into psychic truths.

But what exactly the effect of immediacy consists of and what factors can have such a mutative effect have not yet been adequately described. In order to proceed further with these questions, the dual self-theory proves to be helpful.[3] But these actions of immediacy are implicit, and it takes intense introspection and self-reflection to recognize them.

I would like to use two clinical examples to describe these processes. The first example I take from a paper by Mark Gehrie on the ability to reflect (1993). The treatment described was stuck in a long-standing negative mother transference. The patient had a long history of suffering with a mother who often abandoned her and lied to her. In one session, the patient now urgently wanted to know from the analyst whether he thought she was getting better. Somewhat unwillingly, he agreed with this assessment. Thereupon the patient became furious and in total despair called him a liar: "You are lying, you asshole". The analyst took a while to work through the situation for himself, then said, "I think that when you are so desperate, it's impossible for you to believe me in much the same way as you were unable to believe your mother". To which she replied, "I think that is true. And I do feel desperate". The patient calmed down and was able to grasp the significance of her desperateness both in the past and in the present, and to use it to add to her ability to manage her fractured self (1993, 1095).

Let us look a little more closely at this scene of insight: The analyst agreed a bit reluctantly that the patient was feeling better. That actualized in her an old schema of experience with her mother, which caused her to become upset and desperate. The subsequent interpretation made sense to her because her present despair had a real psychic similarity to her despair at that time, which was now actualized in her in the same way. What does it mean? In order to follow the interpretation, the patient relates the "now" and the "then" in her imagination. This creates an inner affective reaction which eliminates the experience of the time interval, whereby the *affective* content of both scenes is experienced as identical. This perception of identity generates a feeling of an overwhelming sense of immediacy, which can be put into words like this: "This is exactly the same". This immediacy is the first step toward insight. But then the experience of time between then and now becomes virulent again together with an immediate sense of continuity of the self, a feeling that can be put into words like this: "That is indeed me, who experiences that". These are all components of the "pure" pre-reflexive experience of the act of insight, which we must attribute to the agentive self. The inner force with which this act comes into effect shakes the mental equilibrium, whereby unconscious layers can be activated. As I said, these are all pure agency components of insight, which then are merged with the representational parts of the self activated by the interpretation.

I would like to explain the importance of the act by which an insight suddenly opens up with a second example. A 30-year-old female patient had been suffering from juvenile diabetes since the age of five, which had been discovered in a clinic under traumatic circumstances at that time. Since then, she suffered from traumatic abandonment anxieties and got into dissociative states in which her self was leaving her body and she did not feel herself anymore. After about a year and a half of treatment, the patient was about to undergo retinal laser surgery. She started having panic attacks and began dissociating again, a typical reaction of hers when she had to go to the ophthalmologist. She came to the session in this state. She described for the first time details of an eye surgery for strabismus, which had been performed when she was three years old. She still remembered the details of how she was tied to the bed so that she could not tear off the bandage over her eyes. She had hovered up to the ceiling and looked down on herself from above. She was no longer in her body. For me the description caused a sudden insight and I spontaneously said to her: "That was the moment when you started to wander out of yourself and that was the break in your self". The patient reported that my words had run through her like a shock and like an adrenaline kick. The session had an immediate effect. Her restlessness and constant overexcitement disappeared. She was able to get through the laser surgery without much anxiety. She no longer felt split, but more unified. It was a feeling as if a clamp had been loosened inside her; she was no longer tied up by anxiety as before, but had the feeling of expanding. For the first time in her life, she felt a stable sense of unity and continuity of self.

Through my interpretation her current dissociative state and her anxiety became directly connected to the original traumatic situation. The old scene and the present scene had been de-differentiated and experienced as identical. This has abruptly and immediately triggered an emotional blow. The experience of time was eliminated. Patients often express the immediacy of this experience in this way: "That's right", "yes, that's how it is", or "that goes deep". After this experience does the sense of continuity set in again. The temporal distance comes into play again and the circumstances of the scenes are differentiated. The pre-reflexive part of the process of insight driven by the self-agency now passes over into its descriptive-representational experience. The self is relieved of the affective pressure of a pattern of action which has trapped her in the past. A new perspective emerges with a momentary new degree of freedom to reflect and to create a descriptive insight.

I hope to have shown how a dual theory of the self can help us to better understand the moment of immediacy in the effect of interpretations. The agentive self, with its structural power, has a central position in initiating mental transformations. Without its participation, the insights of the representational self would remain limited to a cognitive descriptive level. Richfield (1954, 407), who emphasized the duality in the process of insight, quoted Freud's famous statement, "The voice of reason is silent", and expanded it by adding: "the reason has two voices".

## Notes

1  There are problems with Mead's nomenclature when translating it into German. In German, I and me would actually both be translated as "Ich". The translator of Mead's main work "Mind, self and society" chose the following solution, the "I" he translates as "Ich", the me as "ICH". The "self" he translates not as "self" but as "identity". In this, Erikson's definition of identity resonates, for the self is a process with two distinct phases of "I" and "me". But this solution creates more confusion than clarity in the text. I therefore stick to the concept of self. I sometimes use the English terms "I" or "me" in certain places, but predominantly I translate the "I" as "agency of the self" or use the English "agentive self" which I translate as "das Selbst als mentaler Akteur" and for the "me" I use "representational self" (das repräsentationale Selbst). I thus follow a suggestion made by Fonagy et al. (2002).

2  For more details, see Bohleber (2022).
3  Bell and Leite (2016) revisit the problem of "experiential self-understanding" as a basis for psychological change, but take a very different approach to explaining it.

## Bibliography

Abram, J. (2007): *The language of Winnicott. A dictionary of Winnicott's use of words, 2nd ed.* London and New York: Routledge.

Bell, D. & Leite, A. (2016): Experiential self-understanding. *International Journal of Psychoanalysis, 97*: 305–332.

Bohleber, W. (2022): Das Selbst als mentaler Akteur. Ein vernachlässigtes Konzept der Psychoanalyse. *Forum der Psychoanalyse, 38*: 17–32.

Dews, P. (1995): The paradigm shift to communication and the question of subjectivity: Reflections on Habermas, Lacan and Mead. *Revue Internationale de Philosophie, 4(194)*: 483–519.

Erikson, E.H. (1959): *Identity and the life cycle.* New York: International Universities Press.

Erikson, E.H. (1968): *Youth and crisis.* New York: Norton.

Erikson, E.H. (1970): Autobiographic notes on the identity crisis. *Daedalus, 97*:154–176.

Erikson, E.H. (1981): The Galilean sayings and the sense of "I". *Psychoanalysis and Contemporary Thought, 19*: 291–337.

Fonagy, P., Gergeley, G., Jurist, E. & Target, M. (2002): *Affect regulation, mentalization, and the development of the self.* New York: Other Press.

Freud, S. (1933): *New introductory letters in psychoanalysis. S.E. 22.*

Friedman, L.J. (1999): *Identity's architect. A biography of Erik H. Erikson.* London: Free Associations Books.

Gehrie, M. (1993): Psychoanalytic technique and the development of the capacity to reflect. *Journal of the American Psychoanalytic Association, 41*: 1083–1111.

Greenson, R. (1967): *The technique and practice of psychoanalysis.* New York: International Universities Press.

Hartmann, H. (1950/1964): *Essays on ego psychology. Selected problems in psychoanalytic theory.* New York: International Universities Press.

James, W. (1890): *Principles of psychology.* New York: Henry Holt.

James, W. (1892): *Textbook of psychology.* London: Macmillan and Co.

Laplanche, J. & Pontalis, J.-B. (1988): *The language of psychoanalysis. Vol. 1 & 2.* London: Karnac.

Mead, G.H. (1934): *Mind, self and society. From the standpoint of a social behaviorist.* Chicago, IL: Chicago University Press.

Modell, A.H. (1993): *The private self.* Cambridge and London: Harvard University Press.

Modell, A. (2008): Horse and rider revisited: The dynamic unconscious and the self as agent. *Contemporary Psychoanalysis, 44*: 351–366.

Plessner, H. (1928): *Die Stufen des Organischen und der Mensch. Einleitung in die philosophische Anthropologie. Gesammelte Schriften IV.* Frankfurt: Suhrkamp, 2003.

Plessner, H. (1961): *Die Frage nach der Conditio humana. Gesammelte Schriften Bd. VIII.* Frankfurt: Suhrkamp, 2003: 136–217.

Poland, W. (1988): Insight and the analytic dyad. *Psychoanalytic Quarterly 57*: 341–369.

Richfield, J. (1954): An analysis of the concept of insight. *Psychoanalytic Quarterly* 23: 390–408.

Sander, L.W. (2008): *Living systems, evolving consciousness, and the emerging person.* Routledge: New York, 2014.

Sterba, R. (1934): The fate of the ego in analytic therapy. *International Journal of Psychoanalysis, 15*: 117–126.

Stern D.N. (2004): *The present moment in psychotherapy and everyday life.* New York: Norton.

Strachey, J. (1934): The nature of the therapeutic action of psycho-analysis. *International Journal of Psychoanalysis, 15*: 127–159.

Tugendhat, E. (1979): *Selbstbewusstsein und Selbstbestimmung. Sprachanalytische Interpretationen.* Frankfurt: Suhrkamp (9. Aufl. 2017).

Waelder, R. (1934): The problem of freedom in psycho-analysis and the problem of reality-testing. *International Journal of Psychoanalysis, 17*: 89–108.

Winnicott, D.W. (1965): *The maturational processes and the facilitating environment: Studies in the theory of emotional development.* London: Hogarth

Winnicott, D.W. (1971): *Playing and reality.* London: Tavistock Publications.

# 9 The mechanism of change in the 'talking cure'

## A neuropsychoanalytic perspective

*Mark Solms*

This chapter is grounded in a large body of neuropsychoanalytic research findings which have prompted basic revisions of psychoanalytic theory but it is addressed primarily at clinicians. Psychoanalytic therapy is an *application* of psychoanalytic theory; therefore, advances in our theory necessarily have implications for our therapy.

The neuropsychoanalytic research findings that I am referring to concern two themes: (A) the nature and number of the *drives*, which, to quote Freud (1915a), 'make demands upon the mind to perform work'; and (B) the nature and component structures of what we call 'the unconscious', and especially of the way in which the *repressed* component of the unconscious is constituted and maintained.

Since the scientific justification for the revisions I will outline below is amply discussed elsewhere, I will not recapitulate the research evidence here (see Solms, 2013, 2015, 2016, 2017, 2018, 2021, 2022). Instead, I will simply enumerate the revisions in a dogmatic fashion. On the basis of these revisions, I will conclude with the main focus of the present chapter, namely: (C) a discussion of the implications of the revisions for our clinical practice.

### Revision of drive theory

With the following eight dictums, I summarize the current state of neuropsychoanalytic revisions of our classical drive theory:

1  There are not two drives but many, at least *seven* of which deserve to be described as making 'emotional' demands (as opposed to 'bodily' ones) upon the mind: SEEKING, LUST, RAGE, FEAR, PANIC/GRIEF, CARE and PLAY.

2  These drives are not 'objectless' (Freud, 1915a); rather, they are *intrinsically object-related*. SEEKING is directed towards novel objects; LUST towards sexual objects; RAGE towards impeding objects; FEAR towards dangerous objects; PANIC/GRIEF towards caregiving objects; CARE towards dependent objects; and PLAY towards competing objects.

DOI: 10.4324/9781032651934-12

(The objects are *implicit* in these drives, in much the same way as Bion (1962) speaks of 'preconceptions'.)

3  Drives are not unconscious but rather *consciously felt*. When drives are not-yet felt, they are better described as 'needs'. For example, the body needs energy supplies constantly, but it makes demands upon *the mind* (i.e. the need becomes a drive) only when we *feel* hungry; we need to remain free from danger constantly, but this need makes demands *upon the mind* only when we *feel* scared.

4  'Drives' are not synonymous with 'instincts'. Instincts (like reflexes) are innate *responses* to drive demands. Fortunate as we are to have them, however, instinctual responses are far too simple and stereotyped to satisfy our drive demands in all contexts.

5  Instincts (i.e. what Freud called 'primal phantasies') are not inherited *memories* in the 'episodic' sense of the word; they are adaptive *action patterns* that promote survival and reproductive success, which were accordingly conserved by natural selection. ('Castration anxiety' serves as a model example; see Solms, 2022.) Because instincts are not memories, they cannot be extinguished or updated as such; they are indelible. However, they can be inhibited and then replaced (*supplemented* rather than extinguished) by alternative response patterns, which are acquired through learning from experience.

6  The primary task of emotional development is *learning* how to meet drive demands in the specific environments that we find ourselves in (e.g. in our family of origin and its socio-economic circumstances). This is more difficult in the case of emotional drives than of bodily ones, for the reason that the objects of the emotional drives (unlike the bodily ones) have minds of their own. This makes them *far more unpredictable* than the objects of the bodily drives (e.g. food, water and oxygen).

7  It is difficult to learn how to satisfy the seven emotional drives for the additional reason that they readily *conflict* with one another. For example, the PANIC/GRIEF drive triggers instinctual behaviours which are designed to maintain the presence, attention and care of an attachment object, while the RAGE drive triggers instinctual behaviours which are designed to get rid of (e.g. destroy) an impeding object.[1] Now, whose mother never frustrated them? As Bion (1962) said: 'A good object absent is a bad object present'. (The conflict posed by a realization that the good and the bad object may be one and the same person underpins the whole of Kleinian theory.)

8  To the extent that a child *fails* to learn how to satisfy a drive, to that extent it will suffer from the feeling which announces that particular drive. For example, a child who has not learnt how to satisfy its PANIC/GRIEF drive adequately will suffer from panicky anxiety or from despair; a child that has not learnt how to satisfy its RAGE drive adequately will suffer from 'anger management' issues.

## Revision of the theory of the unconscious

With the following seven dictums, I summarize the current state of neuropsychoanalytic revisions of the classical theory of the unconscious:

1  The unconscious is *not the same thing as the id*. The unconscious is a *memory* system, while the id is the fount of our *drives*. (Consider Freud's famous depiction of the system Ucs. as a memory system in Chapter 7 of *The Interpretation of Dreams* [1900].) Moreover, the system Ucs. is just that – it is unconscious – while 'feelings of pleasure-unpleasure govern the passage of events in the id with despotic force' (Freud, 1939, p. 198). It is commonplace to suffer feelings without knowing where they come from; feelings are *conscious* but the memories which *cause* them need not be. Hence, 'hysterics suffer [consciously] mainly from [unconscious] reminiscences' (Freud & Breuer, 1895, p. 7).

2  Memories are *about* the past, but they are *for* the future. The only reason we learn from the past is to better predict the future. In neuropsychoanalysis, therefore, we speak of the memory systems as 'prediction' systems.

3  There are *three kinds of memory systems*, one 'short-term' and two 'long-term' systems. What Freud called the system Cs., we now call the short-term memory system. This is the part of the ego that performs ongoing *predictive work* in response to the demands of the id. We call this process 'working memory' (which entails actively holding something in mind while thinking it through; it is akin to what Freud called the 'secondary process'). The products of this work – that is, the predictions that arise from it – are deposited into 'long-term' memory. This encoding process is called 'consolidation'. Consolidation is necessary because the short-term memory system has extremely limited capacity.

The two long-term memory systems are called the 'declarative' and 'nondeclarative' systems. They coincide with what Freud called the systems Pcs. and Ucs., respectively. Declarative predictions are accordingly capable of returning to the conscious state (i.e. of being retrieved back into short-term memory). This renders them labile once more. In other words, they become uncertainties rather than predictions. Hence, 'consciousness arises *instead of* a memory trace' (Freud, 1920, p. 25). This memory-updating process is called 'reconsolidation'.

Nondeclarative predictions, by contrast, are *incapable of returning to the conscious state*. They take the form of automatized responses, akin to the instincts described previously. The only way these predictions can be 'remembered' is by them being *enacted*. (They are *repeated* instead of remembered; cf. Freud, 1914.) Nondeclarative – i.e. automatized – responses function in accordance with Freud's 'primary process', and they form the basis of his 'repetition compulsion'. Unlike declarative predictions, which are subject to constant review in consciousness – which forms the very basis of voluntary action – *nondeclarative predictions are indelible.* (They are 'hard to learn and hard to forget', as cognitive neuroscientists euphemistically put it.)[2]

4 Declarative predictions are reconsolidated in response to 'prediction errors' – which are felt because they *fail* (by definition) to meet drive demands. Predictions are typically consolidated into nondeclarative memory – i.e. they are sequestered from conscious reconsolidation, and thereby automatized – only when they meet drive demands *reliably*. This makes it possible to exclude the delay and uncertainty which comes with 'secondary process' thinking.

5 However, some predictions are *prematurely and illegitimately* automatized. This subset of nondeclarative response patterns is called 'the repressed'. Repression occurs for various reasons, including immaturity of the declarative memory systems in the first years of life. (This is equivalent to Freud's 'primary repression'.) However, a more ubiquitous reason for it is the presence of *insoluble problems*, which arise from children's relative inability to meet their drive demands (e.g. the demands of the LUST drive, which present especially insurmountable problems for children). This adaptive limitation of children may be helped or hindered by their facilitating environment. If an emotional problem proves insoluble, the child cuts its losses – it puts the problems out of mind – and automatizes the *least bad* prediction it can come up with. (The fact that we speak of 'repressed *wishes*' reflects their unrealistic and childish character.)[3]

6 Repression results in the situation described above: suffering feelings without knowing where they come from. Hence, paraphrasing Freud & Breuer, we may say: Our patients suffer mainly from feelings. The actual cause of this suffering is the failure of a repressed prediction to satisfy pressing drive demands; in other words, the suffering results from an unconsciously executed, automatized response to an emotional need. These stereotyped response patterns are called 'transference'. However, transference is not evoked in the clinical situation alone and it is *by no means directed solely or especially towards the analyst*. It entails the enactment of childish predictions about how to satisfy emotional needs, which were forged in relation to the primary objects, but which are then repeated in relation to (are transferred onto) present-day objects. People readily have transferences to their spouses, bosses, friends, teachers, celebrities, governments etc.

7 We do not willingly or passively suffer the unpleasant feelings that arise from repression; we institute *defences* against them. This implies that *'repression' and 'defence' are not synonymous*. Defences are secondary responses to the failure of repressed predictions; they are not directed towards satisfying the underlying drive demands (as primary repressed predictions are) but rather towards eradicating the feelings arising from the failure to satisfy them. Moreover, defences are *not necessarily unconscious*. In fact, they frequently are preconscious. (There are

many things that we *can* think about which we *prefer* not to think about. This is called 'suppression', not 'repression'.) Lastly, many defences exist which are not included in the classical lists of the 'mechanisms of defence'. Consider substance abuse, for example: Many drinkers freely admit that they drink to obliterate unwanted feelings (that is why we call it 'self-medication').

## Implications for clinical practice

With the following theses, which constitute the main focus of this chapter, I summarize the current state of neuropsychoanalytic revisions of classical therapeutic technique. I will organize my comments under eight subheadings:

### Two problems with the classical theory of the 'talking cure'

The first problem is this. Freud taught us that:

> It is surely of the essence of an emotion that we should be aware of it, i.e., that it should become known to consciousness. Thus, the possibility of the attribute of unconsciousness would be completely excluded as far as emotions, feelings and affects are concerned.
>
> (1915b, p. 180)

This is the same Freud who taught us that:

> Feelings of pleasure-unpleasure govern the passage of events in the id with despotic force. The id obeys the inexorable pleasure principle.
>
> (1939, p. 198)

This is also the same Freud who taught us that the id is unconscious! The rationale for his 'talking cure', therefore, was that *words*, being derived from perceptual consciousness (from his system Pcpt.-Cs.), and therefore being possessions of the ego, must be dragged down into the unconscious id in order for us to render it thinkable. Hence, 'where id was, there shall ego be'. This makes no sense if the id's drives are consciously felt in the first place. Conscious feelings bubble up from the id, making demands upon the ego to perform (predictive) work; and the purpose of this work is to meet id demands, so as to minimize the feelings we suffer, which licences the ego to automatize its predictions and render them unconscious. The ideal state of the ego, therefore, is *automaticity*: a sort of Nirvana in which we know in advance how to manage all of life's challenges. The mechanism of the 'talking cure' must, therefore, be something quite other than what we have previously thought.

Our second problem is that Freud taught us that the mechanism of change in his 'talking cure' was the lifting of repressions. This was said to render conscious the previously repressed infantile wishes. Freud gradually tempered his expectations on that score and spoke of a 'construction' or 'reconstruction' of what is repressed, rather than a literal remembering of it. But many psychoanalysts, still today, seem to believe that our primary task is to assist our patients to *remember* how they resolved or tried to resolve or failed to resolve the emotional challenges of childhood. I often ask my psychoanalytic colleagues if they still believe that the lifting of repressions is the primary goal of our treatment. Of the many that agree (who say that it is the primary goal), I go on to ask if they still believe that the Oedipus complex forms the 'nucleus' of the repressed. This question, too, is usually answered in the affirmative. Then I ask: How many of your patients get better because they remember how they resolved their Oedipus complex? Do they actually *remember* how they dealt with their four-or-five-year-old incestuous strivings and rivalries, let alone with their earlier conflicts in relation to the primary attachment figure? The answer, almost always, is no. Therefore, in this respect too, we must be doing something other than what we think we do.

My aim in what follows is to replace these two conventional accounts that we use to explain what we do clinically with a set of theoretical propositions which I believe tally more closely with the facts.

### The meaning of symptoms

Symptoms always mean something; by definition, they are *symptomatic* of something. This applies even to physical symptoms. Consider angina pectoris: The patient feels pain in the chest following exertion. This means that the demand for oxygen by the heart muscle exceeds the supply of it by the coronary arteries. This is the mechanism – the *cause* – of the symptom.

However, in the case of psychological symptoms, the term 'meaning' has an additional denotation. It is interesting to note that the core of most symptoms (even physical ones) is an unpleasant feeling; but this is more obviously the case when it comes to psychological symptoms. *Our patients suffer mainly from feelings.* (My children, when they were young, explained to their friends that their father is 'a doctor for feelings'. That is what we are: doctors for feelings.) It is instructive to compare the statement 'our patients suffer mainly from feelings' with the statement 'hysterics suffer mainly from reminiscences'. Psychological patients suffer mainly from things they have experienced which they do not consciously remember. On the basis of what was explained above, we could say that they suffer consciously from the consequences of *repressed predictions* arising from how they managed (or tried to manage) the emotional demands of childhood.

So, to say that our patients suffer mainly from feelings is *the same* as to say that they suffer mainly from repressed predictions. Why, then, should we place the emphasis on feelings? There are three reasons. The first is that the patients are *conscious* of them. Our patients do not say 'Doctor, there is something I am unconscious of; can you please tell me what it is?'; instead, they say, 'Doctor, there is something (a feeling) I am only too conscious of; can you please help me get rid of it?'. This reduces the need for guesswork. (As Freud once said: 'Consciousness is our one beacon-light in the darkness of depth psychology' [1923, p. 18].) The second reason is that it places the analyst on the same page as the patient, and thereby helps to foster a therapeutic alliance. It is, after all, the patient's conscious suffering that motivates them to come to us, and to bear with us. The third reason is the most important one: The *quality* of the feeling tells us *which one* of the patient's emotional needs is unmet. To paraphrase what I wrote earlier: A patient who has not learnt how to satisfy their PANIC/GRIEF drive will suffer from panicky anxiety or despair; a patient who has not learnt how to satisfy their RAGE drive will suffer from 'anger management' issues.

This, in due course, leads us to the mechanism (to the cause) of the symptom. Just as feelings of chest pain after exertion tell us that a patient's heart muscle is not receiving the oxygen supply that it needs, so too feelings of panic or despair tell us that a patient's PANIC/GRIEF drive (i.e. their need for loving care) is not being met. By this, I do not mean that their environment is failing them; I mean that their unconscious prediction as to *how to meet this need* is failing them. This is the crux of the additional denotation I mentioned earlier. When it comes to psychological symptoms, the patient's unconscious *intentionality* is implicated in the causal mechanism of their suffering.[4] (When I first read Freud, I never understood why he said that psychological symptoms give expression to an unconscious wish on the part of the patient. Now I understand perfectly.) So, when I said that the quality of the feeling that a patient suffers from tells us which one of their emotional drives is unmet, it clarifies the therapeutic task: It points us in the direction of what the patient needs to *change*.

But first I want to return to the patient's request: 'Doctor, can you please help me get rid of this feeling?'. There are two ways to respond to such a request. The first is to say: 'Sure, take these pills; they should remove the feeling'. This is *symptomatic* treatment. It is akin to a cardiologist treating angina pectoris with analgesics. The *causal* treatment for angina is directed at its mechanism: It aims to remove whatever is preventing the coronary arteries from supplying sufficient oxygen to the heart (usually by means of a stent or a by-pass procedure). The equivalent treatment for psychological symptoms is to focus on their *meaning*: The cause of the symptom is the patient's utilization of an inadequate prediction as to how to meet the emotional drive in question (the one which is announced by the quality of the feeling they suffer from). The extent to which the public has been misled on this score is troubling: The public is routinely told that psychological symptoms are caused by 'chemical imbalances', whereas the truth is that chemical imbalances (i.e. the neurophysiological expression of drive demands) are caused by a failure of automatized predictions to meet emotional needs.[5]

### The purpose of psychoanalytic therapy

The purpose of psychoanalytic therapy now comes into view: It is to help our patients find new ways of meeting their emotional needs. (Please note: I did not say *to teach* our patients new ways of meeting their emotional needs.) I am not embarrassed by the simplicity of this statement. In the life of the mind, where it is so hard to see the wood for the trees, it is a virtue to have a simple map available. This map serves almost all kinds of psychotherapists equally, but *psychoanalytic* therapy comes into its own when it is impossible for the patient to reconsolidate their pathogenic predictions by merely *re-thinking* them. This occurs when the predictions are *unconscious*. How do we help our patients find new ways of meeting their emotional needs if they are unable, by definition, to retrieve into working memory (and thereby reconsolidate) their old ways?

### Transference interpretation

I said earlier that the only way we can 'remember' nondeclarative predictions is to *enact* them; that is, to enact them in the *transference*. (Please recall that I am using this term in the broad sense in which it was defined above.) Drawing the patient's attention to their transference enactments makes them aware of what they doing, because *they are doing it here and now*, even if they cannot *remember why* they are doing it.

Transferences are generally not subtle things; they are robust patterns of behaviour which are repeated, again and again, all over the place. Nevertheless, identifying the repressed prediction that is enacted in the transference is greatly facilitated by knowing *which* emotional need it was intended to satisfy. For example, a borderline patient suffering from panic attacks is forever finding herself in disastrous situations. The quality of her anxiety (i.e. panic) tells us that this transference is a way of meeting her PANIC/GRIEF drive; that is, it is a way of attracting and maintaining the loving care of an attachment object. This would not be so apparent otherwise. Now, considering the patient's history, namely that her mother only paid attention to and showed concern for the patient when she became ill or was in serious trouble, it becomes apparent what the repressed prediction is: 'If I am in a crisis, mother will attend to me and care for me'. So, the patient constantly brings crises upon her head. She does so even though this is far from being the most expedient and realistic way of gaining the care and attention she craves from the people in her *current* milieu, since they are less tolerant of her antics than her mother was.

This is the obvious shortcoming of all repressed predictions. They were the best (or the least bad) solutions that the child could come up with *then*, but they are far from being the best solution the patient can come up with *now*; if only it were possible for them to re-think them.

This is the aim of transference interpretation. It is not simply a matter of pointing out what the patient routinely does with their objects and what the patient routinely feels about their objects, including you. Transference interpretation is not an end in itself.

It unfolds over four steps, which are enunciated here in a formulaic way (which is not, of course, how we *actually speak* to our patients):

1   Can you see you are doing that (the stereotyped behaviour) over and again?
2   Can you see it is intended to achieve this outcome (to satisfy such-and-such emotional need). [Here it helps to refer to the reconstructed history.]
3   Can you see it is not achieving that outcome?
4   Can you see that is why you are suffering from this feeling?

This *problematizes* the transference. It gives the patient pause for thought; it provides an opportunity for them to re-think the way in which they are going about meeting an emotional need. The analyst can facilitate this process by asking the patient: 'How else might you have gone about that?' This brings the predictive process into working memory, the outcome of which is consolidated in declarative memory, and then – over time – a new prediction is gradually automatized into nondeclarative memory.

### The importance of working through

Transference interpretations that hit the mark are deeply moving for a patient. For the first time, they understand their suffering and they realize that a way out of it is within their grasp. Nevertheless, having just seen the true nature of their prediction, in the very next session it will become apparent that the patient has enacted the very same prediction again. This is not cause for discouragement. It is inevitable. That is because becoming aware of repressed predictions does not *and cannot* extinguish them. All that we can do is make the same interpretation, over and again, as the patient re-enacts the same prediction *in multiple contexts*. On this basis, slowly but surely, the patient consolidates (into semantic declarative memory and ultimately automatizes into procedural nondeclarative memory) a *new* prediction – one which then *co-exists* alongside the old one.

The persistence of the old prediction is the reason why patients can always get worse again (cf. 'regression'); they can always return to their bad old ways, especially when under duress, because the bad old prediction remains available to them, in nondeclarative memory. The reason why the new prediction gradually becomes the 'go-to' solution, however, is because *it works*; unlike the repressed prediction, it actually meets the emotional need that it is intended to meet.

Working through unfolds over three steps. First, the analyst says: 'You did it again', 'You did it again', 'You did it again'. Second, the patient says: 'I did it again', 'I did it again', 'I did it again'. Then, finally, the patient says: 'I *am doing* it again', while they are actually doing it. This enables them to change tack, in the here and now. At this point, voluntary *choice* replaces automatic compulsion. Then the analyst is no longer required. The patient can, and typically does, continue the process of working through by themselves. (This is the basis of the 'sleeper effect'; i.e. the empirical finding that patients who have undergone analytic treatment [as opposed to cognitive behavioural therapy (CBT)] continue to get better – to get *more* better – after the end of the treatment.)

### A note on defence

Given what I said earlier about defence, it is important to note that our patients seek help only when (and to the extent that) their defences *fail* them. Many defences (sublimation, for example) serve us well. The structure of a person's defences determines their *character*; the shape of the ego's personality. Neurotic defences are more viable (more realistic) than narcissistic ones; and narcissistic defences are more viable than psychotic ones.[6] It is the failure of defences that gives rise to the 'return of the repressed'. However, what returns to consciousness is not the repressed *prediction* itself but rather the *feeling* that the defence was suppressing.

Defences typically remain intact in patients who are *sent* to us, rather than those who come to us of their own volition. This happens frequently with children and adolescents, whose defences work just fine as far as they are concerned. Consider, for example, eating disorders and other addictions. It is the parents, or the doctors, who are worried; not the patient. To the extent that a patient's defences remain intact, to that extent *defence analysis* must precede transference analysis.

Defence interpretation takes this form: 'Can you see you are doing this in order not to feel that?' The patient frequently retorts: 'Yes I know, but I *need* to do that!'. Please note the 'I know', which reveals that the defence is preconscious. Patients frequently can think about and re-think their defences.

*It is very important not to confuse defence with transference*. Defence obscures the transference (which, unlike defence, involves a repetition of a *childhood* prediction as to how to meet drive demands), and defence will obscure it all the more if the analyst mistakes it for transference.

Successful transference analysis requires the co-operative collaboration of the patient. Defence frequently prevents such co-operation, and it can readily work against the treatment.

### Three technical recommendations

Based on what I have said above, I will close this chapter with three simple recommendations for practicing clinicians, recommendations which are especially useful at the *commencement* of a psychoanalytic treatment.

To take our clinical bearings, I recommend that we ask ourselves these three questions:

1 What *feeling* is this patient suffering from? (Which *emotional need* is not being met?)
2 What *automatized prediction* does this patient use to meet that need? (This is enacted in the *transference*, broadly defined, and *reconstructed* from the history.)
3 How does this patient *defend* themselves against the feeling they are suffering from? (Repression is not the same as defence.)

The most common mistake is to treat the first task as an *analytic* task. It is not an analytic task; it is a *descriptive* one, in the sense of descriptive psychiatry. Psychoanalysts tend to think: 'The patient says they are feeling *this* but really (unconsciously) they are feeling *that*.' When I speak of the feeling that a patient is suffering from, I mean 'suffering' in the sense of what it is that is distressing the patient *consciously*. *It is usually the presenting complaint* (unless it is obscured by defence; but recall that patients usually come to us when their defences fail). The only difficult part of the first task is for the analyst to become acquainted with all seven of the emotional drives enumerated above. Most of us are familiar with the feelings associated with FEAR and PANIC (we just need to learn how to differentiate between them), and we are likewise familiar with LUST, RAGE and PANIC/GRIEF; but we are not familiar with the feelings associated with CARE, SEEKING and PLAY. However, once you become acquainted with these prototypical feelings, you cannot miss them. (It is like learning to recognize the difference between a chardonnay and a sauvignon blanc.) Moreover, it is important to note that people *suffer* from the so-called 'positive' drives, too. The feelings associated with *every* drive have both positive and negative valences. For example, a patient who suffers from CARE – which is supposedly positive – might feel that they cannot cope with their nurturing responsibilities (consider post-partum depression); or a patient's need to CARE for their little ones might conflict with their other needs, leading to RAGE (and thence, sadly, sometimes to child abuse).

The most common mistake associated with the *second* task enumerated above is to conflate it with the first one. It is only at the second step that we take account of the *interactions between* the drives. This is an analytic task. It is only at this second step that we consider how the main feeling which the patient suffers from arises from the conflicts between their drives. Patients do not suffer from only one feeling, of course, but the single drive that fuels the *presenting complaint* is the one that was sacrificed in the process of compromise formation between the drives (in the process of what Freud called 'drive fusion', aiming for what Klein called the 'depressive position').

The third task is typically the least important one, for the reason I mentioned before: Patients usually come to us only when and to the extent that their defences have failed them.

### Closing remarks

Proceeding in the way I have recommended here is, I admit, not to proceed 'without memory or desire'.

I confess that I do not proceed without desire. I try to help my patients ameliorate their suffering. That is why they have consulted me in the first place. I consider it my ethical obligation to try to help them. When Freud penned his 'Recommendations for Physicians Practicing Psychoanalysis', I do not believe that he considered it necessary to tell his medical colleagues that the aim of any treatment is to ameliorate suffering. He took that much for granted. What he added to the obvious was to tell them that trying *too hard* or needing *too much* to help our patients can have the opposite effect. In other words, *in order to ameliorate suffering*, we should not try too hard or need too much to help.

If you follow my three recommendations, they will eventually become second nature to you (they will gradually become an automatized background to your 'evenly suspended attention'). Then you can proceed 'without memory' in the sense of 'without *conscious* memory'. Everything we learnt in our psychoanalytic training is not *forgotten*; rather, it is consolidated into nondeclarative memory, where it becomes habitual. If it were otherwise – if we literally proceeded *without memory* – there would be no point in undergoing training.

With that said, and having exceeded the word limit imposed on the authors of these chapters, I must close.

### Notes

1 The 'superego', which, as Freud (1923) taught us, lies closer to the id than does the ego, arises from conflicts between RAGE on the one hand and PANIC/ GRIEF, FEAR and PLAY on the other; drive conflicts which yield feelings of guilt, paranoia and shame, respectively. I might as well add here that there are several varieties of *narcissism*. Feeling unloved (PANIC/GRIEF), for example, is quite different from feeling inferior (PLAY) or bored (SEEKING).
2 Not all nondeclarative predictions are hard to learn, however. Consider fear conditioning, which can occur on the basis of a single exposure to trauma. What best characterizes nondeclarative predictions, therefore, is *hard-to-forget-ness*.
3 Repression is the basis for what Freud (1915b) enumerated as the four "special characteristics of the system unconscious". The Ucs. is *timeless* because repressed predictions are not subject to updating on the basis of subsequent experience. The Ucs. *tolerates mutual contradiction* because repressed predictions do not entail adequate solutions to life's problems. The Ucs. *prioritizes psychical reality over material reality* because repressed predictions are impervious to evidence (to

prediction error). The Ucs. *deploys primary process mobility of cathexes* because repressed predictions are automatized.

4   To the extent that a patient's unconscious intentionality is implicated in the causal mechanism of a *physical* symptom, to that extent it is *also* a psychological symptom (e.g., it is a psychosomatic or a 'lifestyle' disease).

5   Of course, there is a place in psychiatry for symptomatic treatment (e.g. to activate the SEEKING drive sufficiently to enable clinically depressed patients to undertake psychotherapy).

6   Here is a condensed neuropsychoanalytic update of the classical psychoanalytic taxonomy of defences. Neurotic defences entail *substitute formation* (the ego substitutes the *object* or the *aim* of the drive in the repressed prediction). Narcissistic defences entail *splitting*, in Melanie Klein's sense (i.e. the ego splits itself and its objects, and projects the *source* of the drive in the repressed prediction; put differently, they project their unpleasant feelings into their objects, and introject the objects' pleasant ones into themselves). Psychotic defences entail *disavowal* (the ego withdraws from *reality*, because that is where 'prediction error' occurs, with its attendant unpleasant feelings). On this basis, they avoid suffering, but at the expense of the very possibility of drive satisfaction – since drives can only be satisfied 'out there' in the world. This, in turn, requires them to create a delusional reality, and then to sample only those parts of the world which *confirm* their repressed predictions.

## References

Bion, W. (1962) A theory of thinking. *International Journal of Psychoanalysis*, 43, 306–310.

Freud, S. (1900) The interpretation of dreams. In J. Strachey (ed.) *Standard Edition of the Complete Psychological Works of Sigmund Freud*, 4 & 5. London: Hogarth Press.

Freud, S. (1914) Repeating, remembering and working through. In J. Strachey (ed.) *Standard Edition of the Complete Psychological Works of Sigmund Freud*, 12. London: Hogarth Press, pp. 147–156.

Freud, S. (1915a) Instincts and their vicissitudes. In J. Strachey (ed.) *Standard Edition of the Complete Psychological Works of Sigmund Freud*, 14. London: Hogarth Press, pp. 117–140.

Freud, S. (1915b) The unconscious. In J. Strachey (ed.) *Standard Edition of the Complete Psychological Works of Sigmund Freud*, 14. London: Hogarth Press, pp. 159–215.

Freud, S. (1920) Beyond the pleasure principle. In J. Strachey (ed.) *Standard Edition of the Complete Psychological Works of Sigmund Freud*, 18. London: Hogarth Press, pp. 7–64.

Freud, S. (1923) The ego and the id. In J. Strachey (ed.) *Standard Edition of the Complete Psychological Works of Sigmund Freud*, 19. London: Hogarth Press, pp. 12–59.

Freud S. (1939) An outline of psychoanalysis. In J. Strachey (ed.) *Standard Edition of the Complete Psychological Works of Sigmund Freud*, 23. London: Hogarth Press, pp. 144–207.

Freud, S. & Breuer, J. (1895) Studies on hysteria. In J. Strachey (ed.) *Standard Edition of the Complete Psychological Works of Sigmund Freud*, 2. London: Hogarth Press.

Solms, M. (2013) The conscious id. *Neuropsychoanalysis*, 15, 5–85.

Solms, M. (2015) Reconsolidation: Turning consciousness into memory. *Behavioral & Brain Sciences*, 38, 40–41.

Solms, M. (2016) 'The unconscious' in psychoanalysis and neuroscience: An integrated approach to the cognitive unconscious. In M. Leuzinger-Bohleber, S. Arnold & M. Solms (eds.) *The Unconscious: A Bridge between Psychoanalysis and Cognitive Neuroscience*. London: Routledge, pp. 16–35.

Solms, M. (2017) What is 'the unconscious,' and where is it located in the brain? A neuropsychoanalytic perspective. *Annals of the New York Academy of Sciences*, 1406, 90–97.

Solms, M. (2018) The neurobiological underpinnings of psychoanalytic theory and therapy. *Frontiers of Behavioral Neuroscience*, 12, 294. doi: 10.3389/fnbeh.2018.00294.

Solms, M. (2021) Revision of drive theory. *Journal of the American Psychoanalytic Association*, 69, 1033–1091.

Solms, M. (2022) Revision of Freud's theory of the biological origin of the Oedipus complex. *Psychoanalytic Quarterly*, 90, 555–581.

# 10 In search of change

## The role of affirmation

*Siri Erika Gullestad*

### Introduction[1]

Psychoanalytic therapy works well – that is now well established (Shedler, 2010; Leichsenring et al., 2015; Leuzinger-Bohleber et al., 2019). A central question, however, still much discussed both by clinicians and researchers, is *how* it works. What is the mechanism of change in the talking cure, as Mark Solms puts it. Historically, psychoanalysis has tended to search for a unified explanation of the curative process. Key articles on therapeutic change bear titles that speak of "*the* therapeutic action of psychoanalysis" in the singular (see Loewald, 1960; Strachey, 1969; Modell, 1976) as if it were a matter of one single principle. To my mind, in contemporary psychoanalysis, we should include a pluralism of theories about therapeutic action (Gullestad and Killingmo, 2020), and in the treatment process, different change mechanisms are typically *intertwined*. Here, I will discuss the significance of *affirmation* in effecting change processes.

### Transference work

Psychoanalytic therapy specifically aims at changing damaging, repetitive patterns of being in the world, like vicious relationships to intimate partners or profoundly destructive self-images – patterns that are not easily changed through cognitive techniques, because dominant relational scenarios are often stored at a procedural level, they are automatized and mostly executed unconsciously (Gullestad and Killingmo, 2020). Therefore, the therapist must identify them indirectly, by bringing to awareness recurring patterns of behavior as these are actualized in the relationship to the therapist. We call this *working in the transference* – main scenarios are created in early dialogues with caregivers are transferred and activated here-and-now. Let me illustrate this with a clinical example.

Eva[2] had been chronically depressed since she was about 16 years old, withdrawing from contact with other people, living with an all-embracing feeling of strangeness. In adolescence, she had serious suicidal thoughts, cutting herself with a knife in arms and legs. When seeking psychoanalysis

DOI: 10.4324/9781032651934-13

at age 27 (she had been in different treatments before without getting real help), her sexual life was promiscuous and violent, dominated by sado-masochistic interaction with quite random partners. During treatment it was revealed that as a child, a neighbor sexually abused her regularly.

Eva came forward as a quiet young woman, almost shy, but with an intelligent and alert look. She entered my office in a most peculiar way: While other patients use a chair or a hook on the wall for their overcoat, Eva wrapped up her jacket and her bicycle helmet into a bundle that she placed in a corner next to the door, almost slipping along the wall before lying down on the couch – as if not really entering the room. During the session, she was lying rigid and immobile on the couch, often clenching her fists, and stiffening her arms, in silence: "There is nothing to talk about. Everything is empty". Her speech was toneless, without color and life – as if to avoid being moved. There was something mechanical and robot-like about her, beyond the reach of humans. It would seem like she tried to ig-nore her feelings and associations – to escape any personal expression, to reduce herself to zero, to avoid being visible.

In the psychoanalytic sessions, I observed Eva's bodily bearing, her fro-zen position on the couch, her stiff body, and the way she clenched her fists – embodied expression of her inner world (Leuzinger-Bohleber, 2015; Gullestad, 2022). I noticed the way she spoke – her voice was monotonous, expressionless, warding off all spontaneous affects. Eva's way of talking and relating was not related to specific dynamic content, to what she was talking about, but emerged as stable, structuralized, character-based aspects of her personality. Certainly, to bring body language and character-based ways of being into awareness is therapeutically challenging. As noticed al-ready by Wilhelm Reich (1933) and emphasized by the Norwegian analyst Harald Schjelderup (1941), in working with character pathology, the Freud-ian method of interpretation is insufficient.[3] Instead, one must describe for the patient how she behaves in the psychoanalytic treatment, calling atten-tion to *how* she relates, commenting on the of ways-of-being (Stern, 1994) in the sessions – a form of intervention quite different from traditional interpretation.

The significance of such interventions has been substantiated through recent memory research distinguishing between different memory sys-tems, emphasizing the importance of *procedural* memory (Clyman, 1991; Fonagy, 1999; Kandel, 1999): The child's early experiences of his caregiv-ers are stored as emotional procedures (e.g., how mother reacts if I seek her comfort, or how fathers respond if I get angry with him) that are often not available as conscious memories but are stored procedurally and are expressed in ways-of-being. That is why, the patient will convey something different about her psychic reality through ways of being with the ana-lyst, i.e., through procedures of interaction than through the content of the narrative. A parallel thought is conveyed by Betty Joseph's concept of *the total situation* (Joseph, 1985). The affect actualized in the relationship to the analyst comes forward as a privileged "gateway" to qualities of internalized object relationships that are not easily expressed semantically.

Thus, current memory research substantiates the priority given to transference in clinical psychoanalysis. On this background, argues Peter Fonagy (1999), the psychoanalytic theory of therapeutic action must be reformulated: The archeological model of insight into repressed, "forgotten" psychic material is no longer an adequate prototype. Rather, to achieve change, the analyst must invite the patient to self-observation – to observe what kind of "dance" she invites other people into. Such theory revision is a good example of a productive dialogue between psychoanalysis and other scientific disciplines, in this case memory research. As recurrent, repetitive patterns are hard to change, treatment takes time. Relational scenarios must be brought to attention again and again. That *intensity* of treatment, defined as frequency of sessions, makes a difference is a hypothesis now to be studied systematically in the so-called *Multi-Level Outcome Study of Psychoanalyses of Chronically Depressed Patients with Early Trauma (MODE)* study, (Leuzinger-Bohleber and Ambresin, 2023, see Chapters 2 and 3) – a research project demonstrating the commitment of psychoanalysis to validate its theoretical assumptions.

At one moment in Eva's treatment, I commented on her way of entering my office – I remarked that it seemed like she was almost sneaking along the wall, as if avoiding to really going into the room. This comment instantly evoked an affective reaction. "I don't want to bother you", Eva said. That I commented on her behavior made her embarrassed – she was almost overwhelmingly ashamed. "Not to bother" turned out to be a main relational strategy – a strategy that protected her against deep feelings of shame. In Eva's life, this strategy originated in the relationship to her mother. Eva was the youngest of five children, and when she was born, her mother was utterly tired of children – mother had neither time nor emotional space for her. Rather, her little daughter's needs were felt as a nuisance. For Eva, having wishes and demands toward other people meant bothering them.

To capture and understand the relational scenarios actualized in the treatment, the analyst uses her countertransference. With an example from Eva's treatment: In the beginning, a main scenario that was played out was one of self-sufficiency: Better to manage on one's own, not expressing any feelings, than risking feeling rejected and hurt! Eva's implicit relational message, conveyed through her robot-like way of relating, was that she did not need me. To be sure, observing Eva's body language was important for making hypotheses about her underlying affects. However, maybe more significant as a source of information were my countertransference feelings, defined as affective responses to the patient's unconscious relational messages (Gullestad and Killingmo, 2020). In response to Eva mechanical way of being, I felt bodily stiff and emotionally bored. More than anything I felt shut out, not being able to reach her – I was "put" in a position of an object that was to feel that whatever I did, I would not be able to help Eva.

Relational scenarios act as dynamic units; the patient casts the therapist into specific roles, which the therapist may become aware of through her role-responsiveness (Sandler, 1976). At times, we are "caught" in the pre-scribed roles and act in accordance with them. During a period in the anal-ysis with Eva, I felt intensely frustrated, irritated, and powerless by not being able to reach her – and my frustration became obvious in some of my comments to her. I became, so to speak, the rejecting object that Eva was afraid that I would be. This *enactment* (Bohleber et al., 2013; Gullestad and Killingmo, 2020) of my countertransference worked, I would say, as a kind of wakeup call for me. I suddenly became aware of the destruc-tive relational drama that I had become part of. This opened for seeing the frightened child hiding behind Eva's robot-like appearance. The use of countertransference as a therapeutic tool, enabling understanding of au-tomatized emotional procedures which may otherwise remain inaccessible, is specific for psychoanalytic treatment.

## Affirmation

What is the mechanism of change in the talking cure? Let me first repeat the core elements of psychoanalytic therapeutic technique: first, identification of dominant emotions, and linking of feelings to past experiences; second, drawing attention to feelings that are regarded as unacceptable and to the ways the patient avoids such feelings; third, focusing on the here-and-now and drawing connections between the therapy relationship and other re-lationships (Shedler, 2010; Solms, 2023, see Chapter 9). The main mecha-nism of change implied is *emotional insight*. Insight into what I really feel, why I find my feelings intolerable, and what I do to protect myself against such feelings, gained through interpretation – in line with classical psycho-analytic theory. We remember how Freud addressed Elisabeth von R., by interpreting her unaccepted feeling, "drily", Freud states: "So for a long time you had been in love with your brother-in-law" (Freud, 1893, 157). Elisabeth was abhorred at this interpretation! Certainly, to profit from this kind of interpretation presupposes a quite high level of ego functioning. To achieve emotional insight with the power of initiating change, interpreta-tion must often be supplemented by another kind of intervention – namely *affirmation*.

Let me illustrate with an example from Eva's treatment. Eva's feeling of shame was at times so shattering that it blocked all personal expression, resulting in long silences during the sessions. Eva did, however, express herself by writing. From early on she gave me written letters conveying her feelings, memories from her childhood that had been activated in the therapeutic dialogue as well as what she wanted to say to me but didn't dare to pronounce – writing acted as a barrier against more direct emo-tional exchange. To begin with, I just described the mechanism of isolating affects: "It seems that you can express yourself quite fluently in writing, but not in speaking. Then you become mute". Such comments were intended to make Eva conscious of the very way she functioned. She became mindful of how reserved and withdrawn she was – until then she had not been aware of how afraid she was of becoming visible. I also, however – and this is my point here – tried to convey understanding of the protecting function of not expressing her feelings directly:

> It seems that as a child, your mother wasn't ready to listen when you needed to talk to her. You felt rejected and alone, and shameful for needing her. *No wonder*, then, that it seems dangerous now to express what you feel.

Such comments transmit *affirmation*, defined as a *communication that removes doubt about the validity of the subject's experience* (Killingmo, 1995). Eva had identified with her mother's view of her as a bothering child – it was something wrong with *her*. Like so many patients, she blamed herself for the harms done to her by others – she felt that something was bad with her very needs. Thinking that she deserved what she got because she was bothering, unlovable, and disgusting, she developed a strategy of psychic retreat – never ever express what you need! *No wonder* communicates that the analyst comprehends her defensive retreat, Eva's wish to safeguard herself is understandable – her protective strategy is an attempt at adaption to an unwelcome environment. The aim of my affirmative response was to convey to her a sense of being understood, thus legitimating her self-experience.

In developing the concept of affirmation, Killingmo's point of departure is what he sees as a need for a broader psychoanalytic conceptualization of psychopathology – intrapsychic conflict must be supplemented by developmental *deficits* (Killingmo, 1989). Specifically, lack of mentalization (Lecours and Bouchard, 1997) is underscored as a significant psychological deficit. Due to deficient capacity to mentalize, "the individual cannot (1) represent feeling states meaningfully in symbols and words, (2) experience affects as his own, (3) relate to himself as an agent" (Killingmo, 2006, 15). It should be emphasized, Killingmo states, that conflict-deficit is not a question of either-or – we all have areas of developmental deficits. The challenge for the analyst is, depending on the "availability" of the patient, to be able to oscillate between an interpretative/confronting mode of intervention and an affirmative mode. Most importantly, affirmation must express an authentic experience in the analyst, it cannot be only a phrase or a technical artifice (19).

To be sure, affirmative responses were most important in my dialogue with Eva. She experienced that I could contain her long silences and psychic withdrawal, which contributed to a gradual softening of her rigid defense, enabling a more authentic affective communication.[4] However, in the treatment process, the affirmative mode was continuously intertwined with an interpretative stance, which at times was more confronting. As I said previously, at one point I felt "put" in a position of an object that was to feel that whatever I did, I would not be able to help Eva – a kind of revenge scenario which I interpreted as such. To my mind, this interpretation was absolute necessary for the treatment to progress. Likewise, when her sado-masochistic sexual interaction with random partners became a theme in our therapeutic work, it was essential that Eva came to realize her *own share* in these dynamics. In childhood, she had been a victim of sexual abuse. Working therapeutically with the abuse provided insight into a pattern of role-reversal: In the sado-masochistic sexual interaction in her actual life, she loved to dominate and frustrate her partners by denying them satisfaction. By playing the cruel, molesting part of her former abuser, she reversed the old roles, thereby getting revenge. As a derivative of the same pattern was realized in Eva's fantasies of dominating me, it was possible to work with these embodied, actualized affects in the transference. My point here is to emphasize that affirmative responses usually need to be intertwined with interpretation, aiming at establishing connections between current and past relational scenarios.

## Affirmation as a mechanism of change

Affirmation emerges not only as a specific kind of intervention but also as a mechanism of change. Discussing the psychological and therapeutic effects of affirmative responses, Killingmo (2006) emphasizes that the experience of being *seen, understood, listened* to, and *accepted* – which is the aim of affirmation – strengthens the inner feeling of a strategic "I". The psychological effect can also be described from the point of view of self-representation. The affirmative response furnishes the self-representation with qualities like *existence, attachment, value,* and *legitimacy,* says Killingmo (2006, 17), aiming at sustaining the self-representation as a stable center of reference and agency.

I would like to consider some of the processes involved in affirmation in more detail, first from a motivational perspective. Recently, Mark Solms, based on new knowledge of affective neuroscience, has challenged us to revise Freudian drive theory (Solms, 2018). By identifying and detailing the basic needs we share with all mammals, Solms contributes to the scientific foundation of the psychoanalytic theory of motivation. Certainly, it can be argued that drive theory has already for a long time been revised since Freud's time, through e.g., the emphasis on the child's primary need for the object, by object relations theory and attachment research, and for self-affirmation, as underlined by self-psychology: Our understanding of motivation must include *relational needs* in addition to sexual drive and aggression. Fundamental relational needs include (1) need for safety, (2) need for self-affirmation, and (3) need for community (Gullestad and Killingmo, 2020).

### The need for community

The need for community is about contact. In everyday language, "contact" and "attachment" are often employed as synonymous concepts. "Attachment" and the biologically based "attachment system" is, however, theoretically founded in survival, safety, and protection against danger. As such, a child may be securely attached (in the sense of having a base to seek out when it needs consolation, protection, etc.) without thereby experiencing "contact". The need for contact, to the contrary, is about sharing subjective experiences. In a process of affect attunement, says Daniel Stern, based on his studies of early mother–child interplay, the parent conveys to the small child, verbally but also non-verbally through sound, intonation, and gestures, that the child's experience can be *shared*. Experiencing that one's own inner world may be shared with another person is a watershed and a qualitative developmental leap – the child enters an intersubjective domain characterized by a "bridging of minds" (Stern, 1985). This is the precondition for *psychic* intimacy. The urge to share experiences – that the other shall see and know what I think and experience – is a deep and powerful motive satisfying an *intersubjective need* (Emde, 1988). It is about a shared "we" – and its opposite is psychic isolation.

### Unrepresented states of mind

Psychoanalysis underlines the significance of needs that are not represented in words. Loss may occur at a stage of development where a mental representation of a specific object has not yet been established (*la chose*, Kristeva, 1987); overwhelming traumatic experiences are often not mentalized but rather characterized by absence (Sandbæk, 2021). Thus, clinically we deal with modalities of mental states characterized by *le négatif* (Green, 1983) – i.e., absence and emptiness. Affirmative modes of intervention may be especially critical in reaching these unrepresented "layers" of our patients' experiences. Through the analyst's attentive listening an event that is remembered, but not represented in its *affective* impact, may so to speak for the first time be constituted as traumatic. Eva first told me about the sexual abuse by her neighbor in a completely distanced manner, without any affect. Through the therapeutic dialogue the abuse, *nachträglich*, became "filled" with horror. Affects – fear, pain, and anger – became represented and "owned".

### Strengthening the "I"

As I stated previously, affirmation contributes to a feeling of being understood, implying that one's experience can be shared by another, thus creating a bridging of minds fulfilling a need for community. By being seen by another, the individual at the same time becomes more visible for herself – "this is how I feel, this is *me*". To my mind, this is maybe the most essential effect of affirmation, contributing to a never-ending individuation process throughout our lives. We don't only have relational needs, we also have needs for "finding" our creative self on increasingly deeper levels – experiencing meaning, not being in relation, but in and by ourselves.

Affirmation aims, argues Killingmo (2006), (1) to sustain an inner feeling of a strategic "I", and (2) to sustain self-representation as a stable center of reference and agency. Thus, he seems to apply two different concepts for capturing the agency aspect of the self. In a recent discussion of the concept of the self, Bohleber (2023, see Chapter 8) maintains that we need to distinguish between these two concepts – the self has a dual structure with a "me" part, referring to the (empirical) psychic content of the self-representation and an "I" part, referring to the agency aspect of the self. "Agency constitutes the vitality and transformative power of the self" (Bohleber, 2023, Chapter 8). It is the "I" that can reflect and initiate change – already the philosopher Jean Paul Sartre (1943), in developing a theory of freedom, speaks about our human ability to *transcend* given circumstances. Such ability is not only something given (as Sartre postulates) but is also a result of development and dependent on a good enough interpersonal environment. Addressing this question, Winnicott (1965) focuses the mother's mirroring of the child's *spontaneous* gestures. Mirroring creates a mind-state of omnipotence in the child, later to be modified, of course, but contributing to a lasting sense of trust in one's own self and one's own feelings (*true self*). This is the basis of feeling able to influence the course of one's life. It is also a basis for personal *autonomy*, which I have defined as the ability to represent one's own interests in situations where these are at stake (Gullestad, 1992).

## Concluding remarks

Mark Solms emphasizes that psychopathology is a question of unsuccessful ways of meeting basic needs, expressed as maladaptive ways of relating to oneself and others. Consequently, the main aim of therapy is to help patients learn more effective ways of meeting their needs, implying revision of what Solms calls action programs. However, this is challenging, as action plans are automatized and typically implemented unconsciously. Therefore, they must be identified through transference work – patients must be made aware of the here-and-now enactments of their recurrent, destructive relational scenarios. This is the essence of psychoanalytical cure.

In this chapter, I have argued that with many patients, an affirmative mode of intervention may be necessary to achieve this aim of gaining insight into repetitive ways of relating to oneself and others. Whereas insight is much discussed in psychoanalytic literature, I have wanted to highlight the significance of affirmation and Killingmo's elaboration of this concept. Affirming, and thus legitimating (*no wonder that…*) the protective function of her massive psychic retreat enabled Eva, gradually, to open up for a more direct emotional dialogue. The analytic affirmative listening to her non-represented affects of rage and pain for the first time, it seemed, made it possible for Eva to experience the childhood sexual abuse *as* traumatic. Increased contact with her authentic feelings contributed to strengthen her feeling of "I", and thus her agency. Consequently, as agency constitutes the vitality and transformative power of the self (Bohleber, 2023, Chapter 8), affirmation comes forward as part of an overall change process.

## Notes

1  A preliminary version of this chapter was originally presented as a discussion of Mark Solms' paper *What is the mechanism of change in the talking cure?*
2  I have previously used the case of Eva in discussing the concept of embodiment (Gullestad, 2022).
3  This focus on *form* has since been developed as a specific aspect of the Norwegian psychoanalytic tradition (Anthi, 1989; Sletvold, 2014; Gullestad & Killingmo, 2020).
4  Patients in the study that Eva was part of were interviewed every six months during the treatment process by a researcher who was also an analyst, and there were three psychoanalytic follow up interviews after termination of treatment (Stänicke, 2010). In the follow up process Eva wrote a letter to me, saying: "Thank you for giving me a new life. I will always be grateful that you saved me from emptiness and distancing, from shame and guilt. And thank you for your patience in endless silent sessions. They were not useless but gave me a feeling of existence. You have given me a deep inner feeling of value".

## References

Anthi, P.R. (1989). Formal defensive aspects of cognition and modes of thinking exemplified by Freud's case history of the Rat-Man. *Scandinavian Psychoanalytic Review, 12,* 22–37.
Bohleber, W. (2023). Self-agency and self-reflection. Building blocks for a dual self theory. In: S.E. Gullestad, E. Stänicke & M. Leuzinger-Bohleber (eds.) *Psychoanalytic studies of change: An integrative perspective.* London and New York: Routledge.
Bohleber, W., Fonagy, P., Jiménez, J.P., Scarfone, D., Varvin, S., & Zysman, S. (2013). Towards a better use of psychoanalytic concepts: A model illustrated using the concept of enactment. *International Journal of Psychoanalysis, 94*(3), 501–530.
Clyman, R.B. (1991). The procedural organisation of emotions: A contribution from cognitive science to the psychoanalytic theory of therapeutic action. *Journal of the American Psychoanalytical Association, 39* (Supplement), 349–382.
Emde, R.N. (1988). Development terminable and interminable II. Recent psychoanalytic theory and therapeutic considerations. *International Journal of Psychoanalysis, 69,* 283–296.
Fonagy, P. (1999). Memory and therapeutic action. *International Journal of Psychoanalysis, 80,* 215–223.
Freud, S. (1893). Fräulein Elisabeth von R. In J. Strachey (ed.), *Standard Edition of the Complete Psychological Works of Sigmund Freud* 2. London: Hogarth Press, 135–181.
Green, A. (1983). *Narcissisme de vie. Narcissisme de mort.* Paris: Les Éditions de Minuit.
Gullestad, S.E. (1992). *Å si fra. Autonomibegrepet i psykoanalysen.* Oslo: Universitetsforlaget.

Gullestad, S.E. (2022). Finding the mind in the body. *Psychonalytic Inquiry*, 42(4), 244–252.

Gullestad, S.E. & Killingmo, B. (2020). *The theory and practice of psychoanalytic therapy. Listening for the subtext*. London and New York: Routledge.

Joseph, B. (1985). The total situation. *International Journal of Psychoanalysis*, 66, 447–454.

Kandel, E.R. (1999). Biology and the future of psychoanalysis. A new intellectual framework for psychiatry revisited. *American Journal of Psychiatry*, 156, 505–524.

Killingmo, B. (1989). Conflict and deficit: Implications for technique. *International Journal of Psychoanalysis*, 70, 65–79.

Killingmo, B. (1995). Affirmation in psychoanalysis. *International Journal of Psychoanalysis*, 76, 503–518.

Killingmo, B. (2006). A plea for affirmation. Relating to unmentalised affects. *Scandinavian Pscyhoanalytic Review*, 29, 13–21.

Kristeva, J. (1987). *Soleil noir. Dépression et melancholie*. Paris: Éditions Gallimard.

Lecours, S. & Bouchard, M.A. (1997). Dimensions of mentalization: Outlining levels of psychic transformation. *International Journal of Psychoanalysis*, 78, 855–875.

Leichsenring, F., Luyten, P., Hilsenroth, M.J., Abbass, A., Barber, J.P., Keefe, J.R., Leweke, F., Rabung, S. & Steinert, C. (2015). Psychodynamic therapy meets evidence-based medicine: A systematic review using updated criteria. *Lancet Psychiatry*, 2(7), 648–660.

Leuzinger-Bohleber, M. (2015). *Finding the body in the mind. Embodied memories, trauma, and depression*. London: Karnac Books.

Leuzinger-Bohleber, M. & Ambresin, G. (2023). Clinical outcome and process research in the MODE-study: From the psychoanalysis of a young man emerging from adulthood. In: S.E. Gullestad, E. Stänicke & M. Leuzinger-Bohleber (eds.) *Psychoanalytic studies of change: An integrative perspective*. London and New York: Routledge.

Leuzinger-Bohleber, M., Kaufhold, J., Kallenbach, L., Negele, A., Ernst, M., Keller, W., … & Beutel, M. (2019). How to measure sustained psychic transformations in long-term treatments of chronically depressed patients: Symptomatic and structural changes in the LAC Depression Study of the outcome of cognitive-behavioural and psychoanalytic long-term treatments. *International Journal of Psychoanalysis*, 100(1), 99–127.

Loewald, H.W. (1960). On the therapeutic action of psychoanalysis. *International Journal of Psychoanalysis*, 41, 16–33.

Modell, A.H. (1976). "The holding environment" and the therapeutic action of psychoanalysis. *Journal of the American Psychoanalytic Association*, 24, 285–307.

Reich, W. (1933, 1949). *Character-analysis*. New York: Orgone Institute Press.

Sandbæk, L. (2021). The relationship between literature and psychoanalysis: Refelctions on object relations theory, researchers subjectivity, and transference in psychoanalytic literary criticism. *The Scandinavian Psychoanalytic Review*, 44, 27–37.

Sandler, J. (1976). Countertransference and role-responsiveness. *International Review of Psychoanalysis*, 3, 43–47.

Sartre, J.P. (1943). *L'être et le néant*. Paris: Gallimard.

Schjelderup, H. (1941). *Nevrosene og den nevrotiske karakter. (Neurosis and the neurotic character)*. Oslo: Universitetsforlaget, 1988.

Shedler, J. (2010). The efficacy of psychodynamic psychotherapy. *American Psychological Association*, 65(2), 98–109.

Sletvold, J. (2014). *The embodied analyst: From Freud and Reich to relationality*. London and New York: Routledge.

Solms, M. (2018). The scientific standing of psychoanalysis. *BJPsych International*, *15*(1), 5–8.

Solms, M. (2023). What is the mechanism of change in the talking cure? In: S.E. Gullestad, E. Stänicke & M. Leuzinger-Bohleber (eds.) *Psychoanalytic studies of change: An integrative perspective*. London and New York: Routledge.

Stern, D.N. (1985). *The interpersonal world of the infant*. New York: Basic Books.

Stern, D.N. (1994). One way to build a clinically relevant baby. *Infant Mental Health Journal*, *15*(1), 36–54.

Strachey, J. (1969). The nature of the therapeutic action of psychoanalysis. *International Journal of Psychoanalysis*, *50*, 275–292.

Stänicke, E. (2010). *Analytic change after analysis. A conceptual case-based follow-up study*, Doctoral thesis (PhD), Department of Psychology, Faculty of Social Sciences, University of Oslo.

Winnicott, D.W. (1965). *The maturational processes and the facilitating environment*. London: Hogarth Press.

# Part III
# Prevention

# 11 Contributing to public policies

## A psychoanalytically informed program for helping mothers and babies

*Rogerio Lerner*

### Introduction

This chapter presents studies conducted with a fast and easy-to-use psycho-analytically oriented screening tool for developmental difficulties in babies aged 0–18 months: Clinical Reference Indicators for Child Development. It also presents a study comparing two groups of mother–infant (aged two to 26 months) dyads: one (high risk [HR], N = 69) at HR for psychiatric disorders in which the older sibling has autism spectrum disorder, and another low-risk group (LR, N = 75) in which the older sibling is typically developing. Infants were assessed for developmental difficulties and withdrawal behavior. Mothers were assessed for depression, stress and anxiety. Quality of dyadic interactions was also assessed. First step was an assessment study with better results among LR than HR. Second step was a clinical trial with HR dyads divided into two subgroups: one (N = 22) that participated in psychoanalytically oriented psychotherapy (12 sessions), and another (N = 47) that did not. Intervention increased mothers' capacity for receptivity to babies' emotional experience, decreased dyadic negative affection and anxiety. Third step was a follow-up after four years of treatment, showing long-term effects. The impact of such studies on public policies regarding early development and autism-related issues is discussed, highlighting the importance of the contribution of psychoanalysis in such domains.

### Clinical reference indicators for child development – IRDI

In 1999, the Brazilian Ministry of Health contracted a group of psychoanalysts and researchers to construct a fast and easy-to-use screening tool for babies aged 0–18 months. A multicenter study was carried out in nine cities. Only a few screening tools for assessing development in early childhood were available at the time, and most were developed abroad, leading to obstacles to their adoption in a public policy program, such as translation into Portuguese, validation in the Brazilian population, training health professionals and paying for copyrights.

DOI: 10.4324/9781032651934-15

Departing from a psychoanalytic standpoint, the perspective that oriented the proposition of the IRDI items was that the complexity of development depends on interactions between maturity and early life experiences, notably with a child's main caregivers. Freud, Lacan and Winnicott are the authors who mostly influenced the composition of the four constructs for the items of the instrument, which will be explained in the following paragraphs (Kupfer et al., 2010).

1  The assumption of subjectivity is the belief of a caregiver that the vocalizations, movements and overall behaviors of their child have some degree of intentionality, although not necessarily conscious or volitive, which is derived from the subjectivity that is assumed to rise in their (child's) mind. Such an assumption is expressed by acts of interaction with a child's behavior as well as caring for and communicating with the child, which usually provides great pleasure for the dyad and is accompanied by joyful manifestations of the caregiver, such as infant-directed speech, also called motherese. Babies tend to react cheerfully, learning that actions have consequences on the behavior of adults and then to repeat the cycle all over again.
2  The caregiver's experience that what their child does is a request made to them (the caregiver). This sets the ground for the constitution of the meaning of behaviors and communications between the dyad, gradually becoming more linguistically complex.
3  The alternation between presence/absence is the contrast between a caregiver's actions that are directed toward the child and other actions that are directed toward other people or objects. It has been stated that

> The mother's absence will mark all human absence as an existential occurrence, which is noteworthy, compelling the child to develop a subjective mechanism to symbolize it. The mother's presence is not only physical but also mainly symbolic. Between the child's demand and the experience of satisfaction provided by the mother [caregiver], we expect an interval, where the child's response may appear, as a basis for future responses or demands.
>
> (Page 36)

4  Paternal function stands for a third instance in reference to the dyadic stance, which is oriented by the social dimension. Being influenced by the paternal function makes caregivers consider cultural parameters in the relationship with the child to limit excess aggressive or sexual impulses and to guide this relationship, while being in charge of enforcing these parameters. The effect of the paternal function is a symbolic separation between the dyad and prevents the caregiver from considering the child as their exclusive "object" of satisfaction. The individuation of the child, the separation of the dyad, differentiation and, in a broader

sense, the interdiction regarding the caregiver's body and words, depends on paternal function.

Both mothers and fathers, along with any person who takes care of a child, are oriented by the four constructs briefly explained above. This is why the dyad is referred to as a caregiver and a child. Some of the constructs are more preeminent in the beginning of life, while others are preeminent later and, since they may operate simultaneously, some items of the IRDI refer to more than one construct.

Constructs are speculative (therefore latent) premises that orient the attribution of meaning to empirical phenomena that are manifested. The items of the IRDI are the manifestations of the four constructs and the condition of operation of their function over the role of the psychic apparatus, in psychoanalytic terms, toward the broader development of the child.

Professionals who use the IRDI include pediatricians, nurses, social workers and community health agents who work in public services and do not have prior knowledge of psychoanalysis.

The IRDI has been validated (Lerner & Kupfer, 2008; Kupfer et al., 2009, 2010) and includes 31 items observed or inquired to the caregiver, expressing healthy conditions related to their bond with the baby, according to psychoanalytic experience and theory. Not all items apply at all times, as they are divided into four age stages (in months), as follows:
From 0 to three months and 29 days:

1 When the child cries or screams, the caregiver knows what the child wants.
2 The caregiver talks in a style that is particularly intended for the child.
3 The child responds to the caregiver.
4 The caregiver proposes something to the child and waits for the child's response.
5 The caregiver and child exchange eye contact.

From four to seven months and 29 days:

6 The child starts to differentiate day from night.
7 The child uses different signs to express different needs.
8 The child makes a demand to the caregiver and allows some time for the response.
9 The caregiver talks to the child using short sentences.
10 The child responds (sound, vocals) when the caregiver or somebody else addresses him or her.
11 The child actively seeks contact with the caregiver's eyes.
12 The caregiver supports the child's initiatives without preventing them from their efforts.
13 The child seeks or asks for help without remaining passive.

Items applied from eight to 11 months and 29 days:

14  The caregiver understands that some demands from the child may be a way to get their attention.
15  During body care, the child actively attempts to play joyfully with the mother.
16  The child clearly conveys when they like or dislike something.
17  The caregiver and child share unique words, gestures or expressions.
18  The child feels uneasy with unknown people.
19  The child has favorite objects.
20  The child shows cute behavior.
21  The child looks for the adult's approval.
22  The child accepts semisolid and varied foods.

From 12 to 17 months and 29 days:

23  The caregiver alternates moments of dedication to the child with other interests.
24  The child bears brief periods of absence and reacts more intensely to longer periods of absence of the caregiver.
25  The caregiver offers toys as alternatives to the child's interests in their [caregiver's] body.
26  The caregiver no longer feels compelled to satisfy all the child's demands.
27  The child looks curiously to things that interest the caregiver.
28  The child likes to play with objects used by the caregiver.
29  The caregiver demands the child to tell them what they want and is not satisfied with gestures only.
30  The caregiver conveys and sustains behavior rules for the child.
31  The child differentiates between objects belonging to the mother, father and the child.

Developed to serve as a fast and easy-to-use screening tool in routine evaluations of babies by professionals who are not specialists in infant development, the IRDI is not intended to have statistical specificity for any diagnosis.

After several statistical analyses (Lerner & Kupfer, 2008; Kupfer et al., 2009, 2010), a cutoff point of two missing items was established: If the dyad does not show what is expected to occur in two IRDI items until 18 months of age, there is a probability higher than a random occurrence (therefore statistically significant) that the child has a developmental problem at the age of three years. For this reason, when the child has two absent items, they are considered to show signs of developmental difficulty.

Two series of development problems were considered. The first type involves the presence of subjective difficulties that affect or are dependent on the child's development, but do not challenge the installation of the psychic [apparatus]. Examples of these clinical situations may be hyperactivity, issues with laws and rules, and enuresis. The second type, also called "problems in [psychic] constitution", covers development difficulties that point out hurdles in the [psychic apparatus] constitution process itself. They indicate more structural problems, pointing to evolution risks that are more geared to serious psychopathologies in childhood, such as global development disorders.

(Kupfer et al., 2010, Page 34)

In a more detailed statistical study, subgroups of items, called factors, were found, when absent, to lead to a significant relative risk of developmental or psychic problems at the age of three years (Kupfer et al., 2010).

## Assessing quality of life at six years of age with a subsample of the previous study: a follow-up

In a follow-up study (Paolo et al., 2015) with a subsample of the previous study, we investigated the association between results of the IRDI applied for children up to 18 months of age and those of quality of life for children up to six years of age, obtained with the Child Health Questionnaire (CHQ-50), which has two subscales: one regarding psychosocial conditions and the other regarding physical aspects. The assessors were blinded, which means that the person who evaluated the children at the age of six years did not know the results obtained in the period from 0 to 18 months of age. Children with two or more absent indicators at 0 to 18 months of age in the previous study had a greater probability (statistically significant [p value = 0.049]) of presenting poor quality of life from the psychosocial perspective at the age of six years.

## A study to evaluate if IRDI is capable of distinguishing between autistic and typically developing children using home videos

In a study carried out between the University of São Paulo and the University of Pisa and Paris 6 (Lerner, 2011), IRDI items were applied blindly, that is, without knowing which group each subject belonged to, to a database including home videos of babies up to 18 months of age; the babies were divided into three groups according to the diagnosis at four years of age: autism, developmental delay and typical development. Home videos of babies up to 18 months old were obtained by Italian researchers when families sought care services at the average age of four years. Studies of children with autism usually use two control groups: one group of children without autism who have developmental delays and one group of typically developing children. This is because children with autism often also have developmental delays, and it is important to differentiate features of autism from those of developmental delays. Characteristics present only in the group of children with autism and not in the other two groups can then be attributed to autism itself. Items of the IRDI have a significant capacity to differentiate babies with autism from other babies with developmental delays and typical development.

Another study (Campana et al., 2015) evaluated a group of babies (N = 43) with an instrument with specificity to detect signs of autism: the Modified Checklist for Autism in Toddlers (Robins et al., 2001). Two subgroups were formed: one group of infants with signs of autism and one group of infants without such signs. The babies in both subgroups were then blindly evaluated with the IRDI. All infants with up to two missing items from the IRDI did not present signs of autism. All infants who had eight or more missing IRDI items had signs associated with autism. Babies who had more signs of autism had a higher number of missing IRDI items.

Results demonstrate that the greater a baby's chance of having autism is, the more intense their psychological suffering in psychoanalytic terms.

Together with the results of the research with the home videos presented above, there is evidence that psychoanalysis, which is dedicated to psychological phenomena, makes an important contribution for the understanding of autism and its occurrence in infants on a group scale. This is critical in detecting early signs and providing interventions that aim to reduce the effects of autism on development.

## A three-step study with mothers and siblings of autistic children

Intervention studies using the IRDI have been conducted on a group scale. The study "Vulnerability of parents and siblings of children with Autism Spectrum Disorder: Characterization of the relationship and evaluation of a pilot model of intervention" was financed by the FAPESP and IPA. It is known that siblings of children with autism are more likely to have the same diagnosis or another developmental disorder compared to those of children in the general population. Mothers of children with autism have a higher prevalence of symptoms of depression, anxiety and stress than those of children who do not have autism. This population has not been previously assessed in Brazil, nor has a clinical trial been conducted to help them.

This study had three steps.

The first step included a case–control study (Durand et al., 2019) of mother-infant dyads with an older sibling that had ASD (HR, N = 69) and were therefore considered to be at high risk of developing psychiatric and behavioral disorders. A control group of mother-infant dyads with an older sibling who did not have ASD (low risk (LR), N = 75) was also recruited. From 2 to 26 months of age, infants in both groups were screened for early signs of developmental difficulties and withdrawal behavior. Mothers were also assessed for depression, stress, anxiety, and social support. The quality of mother-infant interactions was also assessed. In a descriptive analysis, all results were better among LR dyads than among HR dyads.

Statistically significant results showed that up to the age of 12 months, (1) HR infants had higher levels of withdrawal behavior (p = 0.003) and a higher prevalence of early signs of developmental difficulties (p = 0.025) compared to LR infants; (2) mothers of HR infants had higher mean scores for depressed mood (p = 0.008) when compared to mothers of LR infants; and (3) HR dyads had higher mean scores for constrained interactions than LR dyads (p = 0.024). Among the mothers of infants aged 12–26 months, those of HR infants had higher mean scores for intrusion in mother–infant interactions than those of LR infants (p = 0.030).

The second step involved a clinical trial in which 22 dyads from the HR group in the preceding step participated in 12 sessions of psychoanalytically oriented psychotherapy. The results were compared with those of other dyads in the same group (HR) who had not received the intervention. The dyads were blindly evaluated before (no significant differences found) and after the intervention for the same dimensions as in the preceding step. The main objectives of the intervention were helping mothers and babies tolerate emerging anxieties prevailing in their bond; pointing out reactions that tend to make the anxiety even more unbearable; and creating and enhancing more symbolically sophisticated capacities to facilitate integration, communication and the diversification of emotional experiences. Usually, sessions ended up in spontaneous free play between the mothers and babies.

The results showed that dyads who received the intervention, compared to those who did not, showed a greater increase in their reciprocity at the end of the study (p = 0.002). At the end of the study, mothers of the treated dyads presented (1) a twofold reduction in the mean intrusiveness score (effect size = 0.57, p = 0.048), (2) a greater reduction in the mean mother-led interaction score (p = 0.048), and (3) a greater increase in maternal sensitivity (p = 0.019). At the end of the study, babies who received the intervention presented a greater increase in their involvement (p = 0.001) and cooperation (p = 0.003).

The results show positive effects of the intervention, increasing the maternal capacity for receptivity to the emotional experiences with the baby and decreasing their negative effect and anxiety.

The third step involved a follow-up after four years of treatment, in which the HR dyads treated in the previous stage of the study (n = 14), HR dyads that were not treated (n = 18) and LR dyads (n = 25) were blindly assessed for the quality of their ludic interactions, the degree of symbolization during playtime, maternal reflexive function and mental health, child behavior and development. This step was funded by the IPA (process # 3540) and FAPESP (process # 18/03306-7).

Compared to mothers in the nontreated HR dyads, mothers in the treated HR dyads had better scores concerning anxiety and depression (descriptively), had less affective dysregulation (significantly) and had less intrusion (descriptively).

Compared to children in the nontreated HR dyads, children in the treated HR dyads (all descriptively) performed better on cognitive tests, tended to play more with their mothers instead of alone, tended to explore toys more creatively instead of mechanically, and tended to display more symbolic play.

Our results showed long-term effects of psychoanalytically oriented treatment, which may be beneficial for families who are at higher risk of having mental health and developmental problems.

To our knowledge, this is the first clinical trial on this topic using this method in a Latin American country. This work contributes to a larger body of studies using similar research designs and methods that have been pointing in the same direction.

### Clinical vignette from the treatment of a mother and baby (adapted from Durand & Lerner, 2018)

During the initial sessions, the mother's speech indicated a high level of anguish, and the phrases were linked to one another, without any pauses. Although the mother was able to detect what could be of interest to her baby, there was no receptivity to his signals in the sense of "taking [them] in" and emotionally processing them. She needed help to work toward consciously experiencing emotions before being able to work through them.

While the analyst and mother were absorbed in conversation, A., the baby, remained silent, sitting in the corner and playing with some toys, without looking at or calling to either of the two adults. Attentive to A.'s state of acute withdrawal, the analyst says, "When your mom is in this state of mind, feeling very worried and insecure, you become more distant, further away". The baby does not look at the analyst and does not seem to have been receptive. The mother goes on to talk about the baby's motor difficulties and the analyst comments on how the mother felt worried about the two sides, expressing dissonance: One side does not follow the other. The analyst interpreted that this might refer both to the bodily asymmetry of the baby and to the dyad's difficulty in connecting emotionally. Meanwhile, the baby has a cup in one hand, and the other is loose in the air.

The analyst hands the baby a small cup next to his loose hand and the baby, putting them together, starts to knock one cup against the other, looking at the analyst. The analyst is surprised and starts to imitate the baby in his tapping of the objects. She tells him that he is drumming, suggesting his identification with his mother, who is a musician: "Wow mommy, I really like drumming. I like music like my mom!". He seems to truly enjoy this game of imitation, and realizing his intense affective response, the analyst begins to sing songs from her own repertoire. Sometimes the analyst started singing, and he followed, looking and drumming; sometimes he called her to play together. In this playful game, his body showed some newfound organization.

In the following sessions, A. more often established joyful exchanges with the analyst, seeking her out to play hide-and-seek and feeding her "delicious food". The analyst noticed that the mother's gaze and voice were still very emotionally intense, which might have produced a reaction of avoidance in A. Realizing the progressive attunement between him and analyst, the mother says, "Where did you learn these songs? They are so beautiful!". As a professional musician, flutist and violinist, the mother's rhythmic and musical vitality were depleted.

The analyst helped the mother to perceive what she felt and to think on how her reactions to the intensity of her feelings influenced her states of mind and the reactions of her son. The mother expanded the modulation of her voice, which began to be more welcoming to A., resulting in situations of playing together. Mother increased her ability to identify moments of a negative cycle between them, recognizing when A. withdrew and considering this as a defense not against herself but against overwhelming experiences derived from her son's characteristics, then thinking of what could help to open him up to interaction. The sessions favored the expansion of the mother's playful availability, allowing her to recover her creativity, rhythm and vivacity. Little by little, she started singing and making jokes, which allowed the analyst to play a supporting role, no longer leading the interactions. The mother mentioned that she had created a play corner for her baby at home.

## Extending the political scope of psychoanalysis

As a principal investigator of studies on autism, I was invited by the Ministry of Health to be part of the working group to formulate the "Guidelines for the Rehabilitation of Persons with Autism Spectrum Disorder" (Brazilian Ministry of Health, 2014). I was the only psychoanalyst among the researchers who worked mostly with applied behavioral analysis (ABA) and were notably against psychoanalysis. They wanted to make ABA the method that was officially adopted in the Guidelines as the only approach to autism, which would then be imposed on public health professionals and patients in Brazil, a country with 230,000,000 people. Their argument rested on the claim that ABA is evidence-based, while psychoanalysis is not.

I presented an extensive review of the literature that showed that there is no consensus on the clinical relevance, efficacy, or effectiveness of ABA to justify its adoption as the exclusive national official choice. The project of hegemony of ABA was abandoned with the support of the small number of nonpsychoanalysts (speech therapists and psychiatrists) who had no aversion to psychoanalysis.

At the same time, due to the statistically sound published results, the IRDI was adopted as one of the officially recommended tools in the Guidelines for assessing babies considered to have developmental difficulties and more likely to have problems.

Another important result of the work done by various researchers with the IRDI is the formulation of laws aimed at improving early childhood care in the country.

Resulting from the efforts of many professionals, including psychoanalysts, the Early Childhood Statute, Law 13,257/16, was issued in 2016. Among other subjects, the law establishes that the State will provide funds for the training of professionals who care for pregnant women and children up to six years of age so that they can assess their developmental conditions and provide interventions when necessary.

In 2017, Law 13,438/17 was approved, which makes the evaluation of all children during the first eighteen months of life with possible difficulties in their psychological development mandatory in the Brazilian Unified Health System. This is in line with the growing concern about psychological conditions in early childhood and their consequences for the construction of the mind in the most varied functions of development (for example, executive functions, learning, and language), encouraging discussions about the current public policies in various countries.

Since 2021, the Child Booklet, a document issued by the Ministry of Health to monitor and register the immunization, nutritional habits, growth and development of each child in Brazil, incorporates a screening tool for autism (MCHAT). Many items of the IRDI have already been incorporated, and further discussion will determine their eventual increase.

### Final considerations

Epidemiological methods are driven by constructs that are of a different nature from those that guide the psychoanalytic method, which involves knowledge that has roots in clinical work with the unconscious. Considering such a difference is not the same as saying that the unconscious does not impact the constructs that are normally used in epidemiological methods. Researchers who wish to conduct research with psychoanalysis on a group scale can look for standardized nonpsychoanalytic instruments whose constructs are close to those of the psychoanalytical method.

Working with psychoanalysis on a group scale implies challenges that must be faced. Some are epistemological, others are theoretical and some are also narcissistic in nature. There are more than a few psychoanalysts who reject this type of work *in toto*, alleging that it does not consider the psychological singularity of each person and appeals to a scientism that betrays the conceptual bases of psychoanalysis. In psychoanalytic clinical work, psychological singularity is contemplated, whatever the concept on which it is based, which is a different objective (and not contrary, better or worse) of some works addressed throughout this text. This matter seems to be even more sensitive in Latin American countries, where psychoanalysis has been articulated with other fields for ages, mostly in the domain of human sciences, such as political sciences, philosophy and the arts, among others.

Psychoanalysts may or may not work as researchers using methods on a group scale. Nevertheless, they might be informed and able to spread the idea that the belief that psychoanalysis is not evidence-based is no longer sustainable.

## References

Brazilian Ministry of Health. (2014). *Guidelines for the rehabilitation of persons with autism spectrum disorder*. Brasília: Ministry of Health. http://bvsms.saude.gov.br/bvs/publicacoes/diretrizes_atencao_reabilitacao_pessoa_autismo.pdf.

Campana, N., Lerner, R. & David, V. (2015). CDRI as an instrument to evaluate infants with development problems associated with autism. *Paideia, 25*, 85–93.

Durand, J.G., Geraldini, S.A.R.B., Paschoal, L.P., Cangueiro, L., Mamede, D.T., Brito, T.S., Marques, M.V., David, V. & Lerner, R. (2019). Case-contrast study about parent-infant interaction in a Brazilian sample of siblings of children with autism spectrum disorders. *Infant Mental Health Journal, 1*, 1–11.

Durand, J. & Lerner, R. (2018). The link between the body and representations: reflections on a case of psychoanalytically oriented psychotherapy with a mother and baby at risk of autism. In: Brito Wanderley, D. & Gille, M.G. (Ed.) É tarde! É tarde? A intervenção a tempo em bebês com risco de evolução autística (1 ed., pp. 188–201). Salvador: Ágalma.

Kupfer, M.C.M., Jerusalinsky, N.A., Bernardino, L.M.F., Wanderley, D.B., Rocha, P.S.B., Molina, S., Sales, L.M., Stellin, R., Pesaro, M.E. & Lerner, R. (2009). Predictive value of risk signals for the child development: a psychoanalytical study. *Latin American Journal of Fundamental Psychopathology online, 6*, 48–68.

Kupfer, M.C.M., Jerusalinsky, N.A., Bernardino, L.M.F., Wanderley, D.B., Rocha, P.S.B., Molina, S., Sales, L.M., Stellin, R., Pesaro, M.E. & Lerner, R. (2010). Predictive value of clinical risk indicators in child development: final results of a study based on psychoanalytic theory. *Latin American Journal of Fundamental Psychopathology, 13*, 31–52.

Lerner, R. (2011). *Clinical indicators of risk for child development: verification of the discriminative capacity between autism, mental retardation and normality*. Thesis – Institute of Psychology. São Paulo, Brazil, University of São Paulo.

Lerner, R. & Kupfer, M.C.M. (2008). *Psychoanalysis with children: clinic and research*. Sao Paulo: Escuta.

Paolo, A., Lerner, R., Escobar, A., Kupfer, M.C., Rocha, P. & Santos, L. (2015). Association between symptoms of psychic distress up to 10 months and lower quality of life at 6 years of age. *Psychology USP, 26*(3). Doi: 10.1590/0103-656420130043.

Robins, D.L., Fein, D., Barton, M.L. & Green, J.A. (2001). The modified checklist for autism in toddlers: an initial study investigating the early detection of autism and pervasive developmental disorders. *Journal of Autism and Developmental Disorder, 2*(31), 131–144.

# 12 The role of caregivers in the building of self-regulation and symbolization in early infancy

*Clara Raznoszczyk Schejtman, Constanza Duhalde, Vanina Huerin, M. Pia Vernengo and Ines Vardy*

This chapter proposes to unfold a dialogue between the psychoanalytic clinical practice with young children and the findings of empirical research on early development and the parent–infant relationship. Parental subjectivity and psychic structure, unconscious representations, personal history, and reflective functioning which underlie the adult's asymmetrical position in the relationship are in close relation with the parent–infant interactions that are an expression of the bidirectional relational matrix. In this sense, dyadic affective regulation (AR), dyadic emotional availability, parental interactive styles, and the capacity of the dyad to converge and share their experience during the interaction are core aspects of the interactive field. Together with the variables related to parental psychism, its exploration enhances the clinical view and its potential.

Research in the field of infancy and early childhood proposes the systematic observation of interactions as a key tool. Data obtained through infant observational research can work as a resource for the training and practice of psychoanalytically oriented clinicians, as it allows unexpected details that are not easily seen to be discovered, promoting changes in previous knowledge, and sparking creativity for deeper exploration. Indeed, many fruitful concepts were developed by bringing together systematic empirical observation with developmental theories and psychoanalytic practice.

Healthy development takes place in the crossover between the endogenous and the exogenous factors. Sameroff and Chandler, for example, (1975) proposed the existence of a non-linear transactional dynamic system in development in which any one factor transforms the other involved in an interaction. In this spiralized movement, successive encounters between the endogenous and exogenous take place.

The concept of intersubjectivity serves to better understand the complex nature of these exchanges. Intersubjectivity flows between external reality and the interpersonal field, which shapes and structures internal reality and the intrapsychic realm. Although intersubjectivity precedes the intrasubjective, the two influence each other, in permanent co-construction and transformation.

DOI: 10.4324/9781032651934-16

In connection to these concepts and based on research in the field of the infant's sensoriality, Golse (2021) suggests the existence of an innate polysensoriality arguing that infants are born with multiple intersensory and inter-affective channels that will be opened or closed to different degrees according to the unique characteristics of the primary caregiver in the adult–infant bond. Primary innate factors, such as sensory vulnerability and poor sensory synchronization, make the infant particularly fragile in coping with parental and environmental influences on development.

In our research, strongly based on the concepts just exposed, we address the overlapping of theories that privilege parental psychic structure and focus on the asymmetrical relationship between parent and child, such as parental reflective function and theories that prioritize interactive bidirectionality in the adult–child relationship, such as dyadic AR and emotional availability.

## Affect regulation and dyadic emotional availability

Very young healthy infants are receptive to the world and show signs of their own internal activity to elicit interaction and a strong emotional connection with their environment. An embryonic regulatory capacity is present at birth, with individual differences in sensory reactivity and homeostasis. This capacity is initially labile and requires the regulatory and intersubjective scaffolding of the caregiving environment to help the infant develop affective, psychomotor, social, and cognitive potentialities.

Affect regulation could be defined as the capacity to maintain an optimal activation of the nervous system and to control and modulate affective responses. In everyday life, affect regulates our interests as well as our frustrations and contributes to shaping the core of the self (Emde, 1999). As suggested above, infants are motivated to communicate and to co-create intersubjective states with their caregivers. Their affective organization depends simultaneously on the infant's self-regulatory capacity and the regulatory scaffolding provided by the caring environment. In this sense, the Mutual Regulation Model (Tronick, 1989) suggests that infant and mother conform a dyadic affective regulatory system, in which each one transform and is transformed by the other. Since the organization of the system is inherently messy, a co-created relationship emerges out of the ongoing process of matches and mismatches in the mutual exchange of affect expression, and relational intentions. Dyadic regulation enables the child to modulate increasingly complex states of mind and to scaffold the achievement of self-regulation. Parents provide "hidden regulators" (Hofer, 1995) of the infant's states of consciousness and work as affect transformation agents, repairing negative affect and collaborating with the infant's affective self-regulation, expressed by oral self-comforting (OSC) and distancing.

Due to its importance in clinical practice with young children and their parents, we focus on the study of the process of affect regulation and the detection of signs of affective dysregulation observable in the interactions. This allows us to understand certain difficulties in the co-construction of the interactive matrix that contributes to the emergence of the symbolization resources in the infant. In this regard, negative affect and dysregulation signs may be considered expressions of emotional vulnerability. The vulnerability may be present at times of intense separation anxiety, as well as at times of intense pleasurable emotions in which the immature child may feel overwhelmed. These are moments of vulnerability that demand the presence of a sensitive attachment figure in resonance with the child in order to decrease the chances of isolation and withdrawal as a solution to emotional overload. Affective dysregulation in the child, when not satisfactorily repaired by the adult, may have a potentially traumatic effect, may produce difficulties in the processing of stimuli and in the process of symbolization, and may constitute a psychopathological trigger with lasting consequences in the infant's psychic structuring. In preschool, children aggressiveness, impulsiveness, withdrawal, and inhibition are dysregulation signs that can slow down or interrupt the playing display with effects in impoverishing the symbolization process.

Affect regulation can also be thought of from the perspective of Emotional Availability, a concept originally proposed by Emde (1980) and further developed by Biringen et al. (2014) that considers the quality of the emotional connection between a child and an adult involving the mutual emotional exchange, highlighting the importance of the wide range of emotional exchanges that take place between infants and their caregivers including both pleasant and unpleasant ones. This approach also considers the basic principles of attachment theory, which points out the infant's need for presence and contact with another human to acquire a feeling of security that enables exploration beyond the attachment figure (Bowlby, 1988). The adult–infant attachment system accounts for a complex interactive process that is encompassed by intrapsychic processes. The caregiver's sensitivity (Ainsworth et al., 1978), namely the adequate perception of the child's communications as well as the contingent response to them, is a central support for the child's secure attachment to the caregiver which, in turn, is intimately related to the infant's growing capacity of AR. A present, containing, and thinking adult will contribute to the AR and the integration of the psyche in the infant's structuring.

## Mentalization and reflective function

Parental reflective functioning, as a parental variable related to the intrapsychic realm, has shown an impact on children's achievement of affect regulation and symbolic play (Schejtman et al., 2012; Duhalde et al., 2022). Mentalization or Reflective Function, as it is named in the context of our research, has been defined as the ability to perceive and understand oneself, as well as others, in terms of mental states, that is feelings, thoughts, beliefs, and desires (Fonagy & Target, 1998). Along with unconscious representations and parental narcissism, this variable is closely related to dyadic AR as it is considered a key factor to understand the organization of the self and AR. When focusing on parenting, reflective functioning (Slade et al., 2005) is considered an essential aspect of the way parents can understand and signify their child's behaviors. It refers to the parent's capacity to recognize that the infant or toddler has mental states, feelings, thoughts, and intentions of his own and is related to the parent's sensitivity to understand that both their child's and their own behavior and emotional displays are connected in meaningful ways. A parent's reflective capacity allows the child to discover his own internal experience via the experience that the caregiver has of him. This parental feature not only contributes to the infant's increasing achievement of affective self-regulation but also scaffolds the acquisition of the child's capacity to modulate and symbolize affective experience through language.

## Research studies and outcomes

We will present some results from two of our already published studies (Schejtman et al., 2012; Duhalde et al., 2020, 2022).

Mother–infant (six months old) dyads were videotaped in a three-minute face-to-face (FF) interactive situation and in a five-minute Free Play (FP) interaction with toys and were assessed on AR using ICEP (Infant and Caregiver Engagement Phases) Scale (Tronick, 2000) and the FP Scale (Tronick & Weinberg, 2000) and on Emotional Availability Scale (EAS) using the EAS System (EAS, Biringen, 2008).

The ICEP and the FP systems examine microanalytically the mother and infant's expression of affect as well as their affective matches and mismatches and the infant's affective self-regulation signs. The EASs System (Biringen et al., 2014) proposes a global assessment of the affect and behavior of both the child and caregiver through six dimensions using continuous seven-point scales. Adult's dimensions are Sensitivity (affective deployment and intoned behaviors that reflect understanding toward the child), Structuring (adult's capacity to sustain and guide the child in his explorations, and to set limits if necessary), Non-intrusiveness (adult's ability to follow the child without interfering with his initiatives), and Non-hostility (adult's self-regulation faced with negative affect in the child). The child's dimensions are Responsiveness (of the infant to the caregiver in the interaction) and Involvement (efforts of the child to involve the caregiver in the interaction).

The results on dyadic AR showed that in the FF situations, mothers spent 99% of the time looking at their infants, while infants looked at their mother's face 50% of the time. *In terms of expression of affect, mothers showed five times more positive affect than infants and only 15% of the time was character-ized by dyadic positive matches in the FF and in the FP situation. Most of the mis-match states showed the following pattern: Mothers displayed positive affect while their infants displayed neutral affect and maintained social engagement. Matches and mismatches are phases of a healthy interaction.* Although eye-contact interac-tion proved to be crucial to affective development, it is important to be aware that infants are engaged in this kind of interaction for a limited period of time. We sug-gest that the mother's displaying positive affect while the infant displays neutral affect and explores self-regulation resources establishes an enrich-ing path from dyadic affect regulation to the infant's self-regulation and allows the infant to build a secure base for subsequent exploration.

Also, maternal reflective functioning, or mentalizing capacity, was evalu-ated through the analysis of an in-depth interview (PDI R2, Slade et al., 2003) that allowed differentiating between mothers with low reflective function-ing and mothers with ordinary or high reflective functioning (Slade et al., 2005). When relating this variable to the dyadic AR ones, *we found that moth-ers with higher reflective functioning showed less positive affect and more neutral affect toward their infants in the FP situation. But at the same time, these mothers and their infants showed a higher rate of positive affect matches. This could imply that higher reflective mothers can attune to their infant's neutral affect more subtly and accurately than the lower reflective functioning ones* (Schejtman et al., 2014).

Regarding affective self-regulation, *in the FF situation, 21 of 48 infants pre-sented at least once a self-regulation sign, such as OSC, while in the FP situation, only two of 48 infants presented OSC. This means that in an FP situation with toys available, infants displayed much fewer self-regulation resources. In other words, infants at six months do become more object-oriented, showing more inter-est in exploring the outside world than their mother's body or their own. And at the same time, this interest in the surrounding world acts as a regulator itself.*

The high frequency of neutral affect in the infant and *the OSC signs dis-played may be thought of as a message to improve or cease interactions. The par-ent's awareness about the infant's attempt to guide the interaction may help in modulating affective expressions in order to increase the matches.* We also infer that, as mother–infant FF interaction is somehow a stressful and demand-ing situation, infant OSC may constitute a resource for the child to deal with *potential maternal over-engagement. In contrast, in the FP situation, toys and objects are used by the infant to self-regulate and by the mother to regulate the infant's affect as well as to scaffold a developmental shift in the infant toward greater agency and independence.*

The results obtained from the global assessment (EAS) of emotional availability show that the mother's Sensitivity – her ability to accurately read the infant's affective cues and show a genuine positive affective connection – is related to both more positive affect and less negative affect in the infant as measured by the microanalysis (ICEP). Also, these findings tend to express a convergent validity between these two observational sys-tems (global and microanalysis) focused on mother–infant AR.

Another outcome that should be mentioned is that infants use fewer self-regulation (ICEP) resources when mothers are more sensitive (EAS). *Pleasurable interaction, when the infant's affective needs are met, positive affect is present, and negative affect is well-integrated, could work as an affective regulator by itself. In this sense, through videotaped material, crucial differences can be observed between a self-regulation display linked to a healthy autoerotic structure and signs of a stronger defensive self-regulation with the risk of withdrawal in the infant.*

As children grow up, their capacity for AR is transformed and becomes more complex. Children's interactive play is a privileged scenario where affects, and symbolization as an affect regulator, take place. We examined these variables and their relation to maternal reflective functioning in a study where 30 children aged four to five years old and their mothers were videotaped in a 15-minute interactive play situation codified each 20 seconds. We assessed the dyad's mode of interaction (convergent or divergent), the child's level of symbolization (functional play and simple or complex symbolic play), the maternal interactive style, and the presence of affective dysregulation signs, using the Observational System of Interactive Play designed by our team (Schejtman et al., 2012, 2014; Huerin et al., 2021).

*As regards AR, it is interesting to point out that we found significantly more signs of affective dysregulation in the children of mothers with low reflective functioning.* Also, dysregulation signs present a negative relation with the convergent interactive mode (adult and child share the same play agenda) and the level of symbolization of the child during play.

*Another interesting finding was that the frequency of affective dysregulation signs, such as impulsiveness and interruption of the symbolic display in the interactive play, was higher in children whose mothers showed low Maternal Reflective Functioning. Also, children who presented a higher frequency of dysregulation signs showed more functional play and less complex symbolic play.*

The low reflective maternal function was especially linked to mothers' responses to the question about whether they sometimes get angry with their children and how they cope with this anger and with their children's states of upset. Low reflective responses on these items were more frequent in mothers who showed a more restrictive (intrusive-directive) style during dyadic interaction with their children. *It could be inferred that less reflective mothers present more difficulties to perceive and deal with the aggressiveness/impulsivity of their children and, to a certain extent, fail to perceive the discomfort as a message and to offer mentalizing responses to it (Schejtman, 2018).*

## Implications for psychoanalytic theory and clinical practice in early infancy

The outcomes of the studies presented above are in line with a conception of a less idealized early mother–infant interaction than the one that conceives the primary dyad as highly synchronized and characterized by the predominant display of mutual positive affect. Early interaction is an interplay between matches and mismatches that, when dyadic regulation and self-regulation are balanced, allows the baby to cope with the presence–absence of the primary caregiver and the separation anxiety. As Harrison (2022) pointed out in the discussion of this paper, the infant's development of self-regulation, which is essential to creative and productive activity, is linked to the child's emerging internal symbolic representations of the self through the co-creative meaning-making of self and other within the caregiving relationship.

The ages explored in these studies – six months old and four to five years old – are critical ones regarding the differentiation process and the mutual transformational affect changes and are related to the main concepts involved in our research. Around at six months of age, there is a shift from dyadic AR to infant self-regulation. As expressed above, in our healthy sample in a free-play situation only two of 48 infants were engaged in OSC, such as sucking their fingers, while in the FF situation, almost half of the babies presented such behaviors. Then, we may infer that the presence of these behaviors in dyadic play with toys could be understood as a signal of self-exploration that helps to establish a first distance from the mother and shows the baby's desire for seeking or pausing interaction. At this age, toys or other inanimated objects, as a resource of self-regulation, contribute organizing subjectivity. *From a psychoanalytical perspective, we may suggest that self-regulatory resources are related to a structuring autoeroticism that helps the infant to bind surplus arousal during the short necessary maternal distancing, preparing him to metabolize the periods of caregiver's absence and to cope with separation anxiety.* In the same vein, Christine Anzieu (2022) associates the autoerotic creative healthy capacities in the baby with the fantasy of plenitude during the mother's absence. In contrast, she suggests that compulsive, self-soothing behavior can lead to fetishistic and addictive behaviors.

We suggest that when the infant is self-engaged with toys or other inanimate objects, exploring or sucking on them in the presence of a libidinally connected, responsive, non-hostile, and non-intrusive caregiver, a healthy passage from a dyadic regulation to self-regulation takes place. Conversely, when the caregiver is emotionally distant or intrusive and the infant shows frequent signs of OSC and rejects the caregiver's interactive proposal, the dyadic connection may be interrupted with risks of infant withdrawal.

Sometimes even very dedicated mothers find it difficult to tolerate the infant's absence of immediate response and impose their presence without perceiving the communicative signals of the infant, who seeks self-exploration. This is observed in dyads with babies suffering communication disturbances, mainly in the autistic spectrum (Keren, 2022) or in deaf children (Huerin, 2022).

Based on our studies, *we address the relevance of being aware of the inevitable moments of child disengagement and the importance of adult involvement in repairing negative affect and repeated mismatches. This is connected to the fact that the infant's developing capacity to tolerate increasing levels of emotional intensity, be positive or negative, lowers the effects of extreme vulnerability. The extreme sensitivity of infants toward internal and external stimuli may lead them to develop a protective envelope.* The adult is part of the infant's protective system and his capacity to transform and repair negative affects may diminish the potentiality of overwhelming and threatening early affects. The parent's psychic structure and unconscious conflicts, sensitivity, and reflective functioning have a strong impact on this crucial parental function.

*In this regard, environmental failure in building connections and in repairing negative affects may produce emotional pain, and deep anxiety of loss, and may result in physical, emotional, and mental developmental impairment as well as a defensive closure toward the outside world. The protective envelope may then become a rigid shield.* We can consider these circumstances as maladaptive affect regulation, and there is a proven link between these early experiences and severe personality disorders (Beutel et al., 2020; Clarkin et al., 2020; Schejtman, 2020).

From a clinical point of view, we underline the importance of discriminating in the infant a more defensive self-exploration and OSC, linked to withdrawal from the display of self-regulatory engagement, as a resource for reparation of negative affect. This one implies a healthy autoerotic self-regulated resource and a message to the adult to regulate the interaction. *These findings, therefore, offer strong support for the desirability of detection of the early presence of partial withdrawal and rigid defenses in normal development related to parental intrusiveness or low emotional availability aiming to produce early clinical interventions.* The described dynamic, observed in normal development, may have a crucial impact on psychic structure and development, especially in today's intense exposure to electronic screen devices in young children as a way in which parents deal with the difficulties to manage affective dysregulation in their kids.

The parental reflective function, as seen in the second study above mentioned, proves to be a strong tool to amplify parental resources to deal with the daily challenges around the achievement of AR and its influence on the symbolization process.

Regarding four to five years old children, our findings show that the high frequency of dysregulation signs is related to less frequency of complex symbolic play. The adult convergent symbolizing offer in interactive play is central to enriching the child's proposal, adding complexity, and promoting a higher level of symbolic play. If the adult does not perceive nor appreciate the proposal, the child may feel disengaged, with risks of withdrawal, slowing the co-construction process of symbolic complexity. *Moreover, low-reflective parents may fail to interpret the child's dysregulated behavior as a challenging expression to seek self-affirmation and may respond intrusively or critically. In such a case, two paths are possible: Retraction and inhibition of complex symbolic play or defensive opposition, stubborn tantrums, and dysregulation, which can lead to behavior disorders or attention disorders.*

Parents' reflective capacity does not imply the immediate resolution of conflicts, but rather the possibility of containing the emotional impact of the child's dysregulation, linking their own affect with their state of mind and, thus, giving a reflective response to the child's emotional state, instead of responding immediately and impulsively.

Regarding the interactive playing display, in a previous study (Duhalde et al., 2022), we observed that the convergent mode of interaction, in which parent and child mutually enrich the play proposal, was associated with a higher frequency of complex symbolic play, while the divergent mode of interaction, in which a common play agenda is not achieved, was associated with a higher presence of functional play; that is, a non-symbolic play. This reaffirms the conceptualization of the contribution of a fluid bidirectional intersubjective exchange to the unfolding of symbolization, which is a crucial capacity in child's development.

In turn, we have distinguished two types of divergence: One presents dysregulation, while the other doesn't. The delimitation of these two modes of divergence allows us to further understand playing dynamics, and the fluctuation between convergence and divergence states, that accounts for the nature of any relationship, which includes matches and mismatches. A more detailed assessment based on this categorization allowed us to observe that when, in a divergent situation, the dyad manages to resume a state of convergence by negotiation without dysregulation, the play continues and is enriched by the contribution of each member of the dyad. *These findings are useful for clinicians, since the early detection of interactive mismatches and not sufficiently repaired dysregulation is also related to the restrictive parental style, and early interventions on the moment-to-moment interaction may have a preventive impact.*

Finally, our findings brought us to develop changes in our clinical practice suggesting a multidimensional model that articulates the intersubjective parents–child approach with an intrapsychic approach with the child and with the parents.

In intersubjective clinical interventions in early childhood, we suggest that the analyst plays an active role in amplifying affects moving from being part of a new dance between the parents and their baby to remaining on the margins while the dyad or triad unfolds its interactive play. This position lead us to identify the particular separation anxieties of the infant and the regulatory resources that the parents deploy to cope with affective dysregulation. With the parents, we focus on the parent's own history and unconscious conflicts regarding parenthood and on the recognition of a link between the infant's mental states and their own behavior in order to develop new mental capacities in everyday life with their kids. Brief clinical early interventions may have a critical impact in enriching the growing infant's capacity to deal with increasing levels of emotional intensity – positive and negative – to be able to build meaningful, close, relationships.

We suggest that a flexible and multidimensional clinical approach that moves from interactive sessions to sessions with the parents or with the child alone can lead to a deeper and more comprehensive approach to early psychic suffering that has a strong impact on the prevention of future more severe pathologies.

Awareness of early psychic suffering is today at the center of mental health policies, and psychoanalysis has contributed significantly to discovering the early psychic foundations of development. Bridging our theories with results offered by microanalytical observation and global observation instruments provides a very powerful path for training clinicians in early intervention with a psychoanalytic perspective.

The current members of the research team (University of Buenos Aires) directed by Clara Raznoszczyk Schejtman and co-directed by Constanza Duhalde are: Vanina Huerin, María Pía Vernengo, Inés Vardy, Milagros Maurette, Paula Adelardi, Malvina Escalera, Federico Bernao and Sandra Casabianca.

## References

Ainsworth, M. D. S., Blehar, M. C., Waters, E., & Wall, S. (1978). *Patterns of Attachment: A Psychological Study of the Strange Situation*. Hillsdale, NJ: Erlbaum.

Anzieu, C. (2022). Early Depressions: Loss of Liveliness, Withdrawal, Psychosomatic Issues and Risk of Developmental Delay. In M. Leuzinger-Bohleber, G. Ambresin, T. Fischmann, & M. Solms (Eds.), *Early Depressions. On the Dark Side of Chronic Depression: Psychoanalytic, Social-cultural and Research Approaches* (pp. 112–120). London: Routledge.

Bowlby, J. (1988). *A Secure Base: Parent-Child Attachment and Healthy Human Development*. New York: Basic Books.

Beutel, M., Greenberg, L., & Lane, R. (2020). Emotions in Psychodynamic Process and Outcome Research. In M. Leuzinger-Bohleber, M. Solms, & S. E. Arnold (Eds.), *Outcome Research and the Future of Psychoanalysis. Clinicians and Researchers in Dialogue* (pp. 206–215). London: Routledge.

Biringen, Z. (2008). *The Emotional Availability (EA) Scales Manual*, 4th Edn. Boulder, CO: International Center for Excellence in Emotional Availability.

Biringen, Z., Derscheid, D., Vliegen, N., Closson, L., & Easterbrooks, M. A. (2014). Emotional Availability (EA): Theoretical Background, Empirical Research Using the EA Scales and Clinical Implications. *Developmental Review*, 34, 114–167.

Clarkin, J., Maxwell, R., & Sowislo, J. (2020). Comparative Psychotherapy Research Focused on the Treatment of Borderline Personality Disorder. In M. Leuzinger-Bohleber, M. Solms, & S. E. Arnold (Eds.), *Outcome Research and the Future of Psychoanalysis. Clinicians and Researchers in Dialogue* (pp. 174–187). London: Routledge.

Duhalde, C., Huerin, V., Vernengo, M. P., Barreyro, J. P., & Schejtman, C. (2022). Estudio de observación sistemática de la interacción lúdica y su relación con el discurso parental. In C. R. Schejtman (Ed.), *Primera Infancia y Psicoanálisis II: Investigación-Clínica-Prevención* (pp. 163–180). Buenos Aires: Akadia Ed.

Duhalde, C., Huerin, V., Vernengo, M. P. Vardy, I., & Schejtman, C (2020). "Study on Affective Regulation, Dyadic Emotional Availability and Maternal Self-Esteem". Final research report. International Psychoanalytic Association, Research Advisory Board.

Emde, R. N. (1980). Emotional Availability: A Reciprocal Reward System for Infants and Parents with Implications for Prevention of Psychosocial Disorders. In P. M. Taylor (Ed.), *Parent–Infant Relationships* (pp. 87–115). Orlando, FL: Grune & Stratton.

Emde, R. N. (1999). Moving Ahead: Integrating Influences of Affective Processes for Development and for Psychoanalysis. *International Journal of Psychoanalysis,* 80(2), 317–339.

Fonagy, P., & Target, M. (1998). Mentalization and the Changing Aim of Child Psychoanalysis. *Psychoanalytic Dialogues,* 8, 87–114.

Golse, B. (2021). *Mi combate por los niños autistas.* Buenos Aires: Miño y Dávila.

Harrison, A. (2022). *Discussion Presented at the Joseph Sandler Conference,* Oslo, Norway.

Hofer, M. A. (1995). Hidden Regulators: Implications for a New Understanding of Attachment, Separation and Loss. In S. Goldberg, R. Muir, & J. Kerr (Eds.), *Attachment Theory: Social Development and Clinical Perspectives* (pp. 203–230). Hillsdale, New Jersey: The Analytic Press.

Huerin, V. (2022). Reflexiones sobre interacciones adulto-niño en el campo de la discapacidad. Regulación afectiva y construcción de la simbolización en niños sordos. In C. R. Schejtman (Ed.), *Primera Infancia y Psicoanálisis II: Investigación-Clínica-Prevención* (pp. 214–218). Buenos Aires: Akadia Ed.

Huerin, V., Duhalde, C., Vernengo, P., & Schejtman, C. R. (2021). *Manual del sistema de observación de la interacción lúdica adulto-niño – SdOIL. Revisión 2021* (Observational System of Interactive Play-OSIP, Coding Manual, 2021 Revision). Non-published manuscript. Buenos Aires: Facultad de Psicología, Universidad de Buenos Aires.

Keren, M. (2022). Diagnosticar síntomas clínicos en bebés: ¿por qué y cómo? In C. R. Schejtman (Ed.), *Primera infancia y psicoanálisis II: Investigación- Clínica- Prevención* (pp. 269–280). Buenos Aires: Akadia Ed.

Sameroff, A. J., & Chandler, M. J. (1975). Reproductive Risk and the Continuum of Caretaking Casualty. In F. D. Horowitz, M. Hetherington, S. Scarr-Salapatek, & G. Siegel (Eds.), *Review of Child Development Research* (Vol. 4, pp. 187–244). Chicago, IL: University of Chicago Press.

Schejtman, C. R. (2018). *Función Materna. Relación entre variables intrapsíquicas y variables interactivas observacionales* [Doctoral Thesis]. Facultad de Psicología, UBA.

Schejtman, C. R. (2020). Discussion from a Clinical Perspective. In M. Leuzinger-Bohleber, M. Solms, S. E. Arnold (Eds.), *Outcome Research and the Future of Psychoanalysis. Clinicians and Researchers in Dialogue* (pp. 216–226). London: Routledge.

Schejtman, C. R., Huerin, V., & Duhalde, C. (2012). A Longitudinal Study of Dyadic and Self-Affective Regulation and Its Link with Maternal Reflective Functioning along the First 5 Years of Life. *The Signal,* 20(2), 6–9.

Schejtman, C. R., Huerin, V., Vernengo, M. P., Esteve, M. J., Silver, R., Vardy, I., Laplacette, J. A, & Duhalde, C. (2014). Regulación afectiva, procesos de simbolización y subjetividad materna en el juego madre-niño. *Revista de Psicoanálisis de la Asociación Psicoanalítica de Madrid,* 71, 3–24.

Slade, A., Aber, J., Berger, B., Bresgi, I., & Kaplan, M. (2003). PDI-R2. *Parent Development Interview Revised*. Privileged communication. Yale University, New Haven, CT.

Slade, A., Bernbach, E., Grienenberger, J., Wohlgemuth Levy, D., & Locker, A. (2005). *Addendum to Reflective Functioning Scoring Manual – For Use with the Parent Developmental Interview, Version 2.0*. New York: City University.

Tronick, E. Z. (1989). Emotions and emotional communication in infants. *American Psychologist, 44*, 112–119.

Tronick, E. Z. (2000). *Free Play Scale*. Non-published Manuscript. Massachusetts: Harvard University.

Tronick, E. Z., & Weinberg, M. K. (2000). *ICEP - Infant Caregiver Engagement Phases Scale*. Non-published Manuscript. Boston, MA: Children's Hospital and Harvard Medical School.

# 13 "Building Baby Brains".
# A psychoanalytically inspired training program for helping mothers and their babies in Pakistan

*Alexandra M. Harrison and Elizabeth J. Levey*

## Introduction

A lady health worker (LHW) in rural Pakistan visited a mother feeding her six-month-old infant. Her two-year-old child was demanding attention, and the mother was pregnant with her third child. She told the LHW, "I just can't do this." The LHW asked, "Where is your family?" The mother explained that her husband had to take a job far away and could only visit the family episodically, and she and her mother-in-law had an argument and were now estranged. The LHW had taken the Building Baby Brains (BBB) training and was aware of the negative effect of maternal stress on the developing child. She left the mother and proceeded to the home of the mother-in-law, in the same village. "Do you want healthy grandchildren?!" she asked the woman. "If you do, you must go and help your daughter-in-law. She cannot bring up those children on her own." In the next visit, the LHW discovered that the mother and her mother-in-law had reconciled, they were both caring for the children, and the family environment was less stressed.

Providing psychological as well as physical safety to a mother and facilitating her sensitive responsiveness to her infant can produce positive change in stressed families. We offer a method of change through training community health workers in infant parent mental health and giving them tools to enhance maternal responsivity and sensitivity. In our focus on the caregiving relationship, we build on a long tradition of psychoanalytic thinkers, writers, and researchers interested in early development and in particular the infant-caregiver relationship as a port of entry into growing mental health and resiliency.

## Background

While Freud emphasized the influence of early childhood experiences on shaping adult personality, he asserted that an important gap remained in the understanding gained by the combination of direct observation of children and retrospective data from adult analyses (Hartmann, 1950). Anna

DOI: 10.4324/9781032651934-17

Freud and Dorothy Burlingham contributed to this understanding with their important work in the Hampstead War Nurseries (Midgely, 2007). Informed by his pediatric practice as well as his analytic work, Winnicott famously stated, "There is no such thing as an infant," meaning "without a mother" (1945, p. 39). Other early analytic writers – perhaps foremost Selma Fraiberg in her famous paper about "ghosts in the nursery" – described how mothers' behavior toward their children could be affected by the "ghosts" from their own childhood (Fraiberg & Adelman, 1975). The knowledge gap referred to by Freud has now been narrowed considerably by infant researchers, beginning in the late 20th century through today (Beebe, 2012; Beeghly, 2016; Lyons-Ruth, 1998; Sander, 2014; Stern 1985; Tronick, 1989). These writers have contributed to the psychoanalytic literature by explaining how a responsive caregiving relationship supports healthy child development, whereas stress in the caregiving relationship can have the opposite effect.

Environmental stress originates both in material factors such as chronic poverty and poor physical health and in relational factors such as unresponsive or insensitive caregiving, especially in early life. Not surprisingly, these two domains of environmental stress are often linked. We now know that exposure to toxic levels of stress early in life has a significant impact on physical and mental health throughout the life course (Felitti et al., 1998). The infant caregiver relationship is known to moderate the harmful effects of environmental stress during early life, when the nervous system is growing most rapidly. Supporting early development provides the foundation for a healthy social-emotional growth trajectory for the child.

Perinatal home visiting interventions have been shown to decrease violence in the home and improve caregiving sensitivity, which is associated with fewer developmental and behavioral problems in children. In Pakistan, the LHW system provides home visits to families with children under age five with the goal of decreasing child morbidity and mortality. Training these LHWs to support the infant-caregiver relationship offers a scalable approach to early intervention. The BBB program aims to build capacity in LHWs with the long-term goal of helping LHWs strengthen infant resiliency through supporting the infant-parent relationship. The project includes the development of the BBB curriculum, delivering the curriculum to LHWs, and implementing an outcome study to assess the efficacy of the program. Initial findings indicate the need for relationship-focused training for LHWs and for families, while also highlighting the importance of working with the whole family.

### Supporting child caregivers

Supporting Child Caregivers Inc. is a non-profit organization based in the US. It was founded by a child psychiatrist and has as its aim providing support to child caregivers, including parents and others, in various health-care and institutional settings around the world. A current focus has been collaborating with the Health Department of South Punjab and Nishtar Medical University to build capacity in LHWs by providing the BBB 25-hour training. BBB is designed to support neurodevelopment in infants growing up in rural Pakistan, who suffer long-term health consequences from exposure to adverse childhood experiences (ACEs) that stem from chronic poverty and societal and family disruption (Anda et al., 2006; Felitti et al., 1998). Exposure to ACEs is a risk factor for a number of chronic conditions with adult onset, including cardiovascular diseases, metabolic disorders, cancer, mental health disorders, and substance abuse disorders (Hughes et al., 2017; Monnat & Chandler, 2015; Shonkoff et al., 2012). ACEs are highly comorbid, and their impact is additive; the greater the number of ACEs the child experiences, the greater the negative consequences for their adult health. Accumulating evidence suggests that supporting the infant-parent relationship can moderate the harmful effects of environmental stress on the developing nervous system (Beeghly et al., 2016; Perry, 2019; Sroufe, 2009). Neurodevelopment is occurring most rapidly during the period from pregnancy through the first 1,000 days of life. For this reason, it is critical to target infancy, as later development builds on what is achieved during this period.

### Lady health worker system in Pakistan

Since Pakistan became an independent country in 1947, there has been persistent violence and political unrest. A quarter of the population lives in poverty, and Pakistan's under-five mortality rate is 67 deaths per 1,000 live births, the 22nd highest out of 193 countries worldwide (World Bank, 2019), and 37% of children experience stunting, severe growth restriction associated with malnutrition (UNICEF, 2021). The LHW system was introduced in 1993 to address high rates of infant morbidity and mortality by increasing access to prenatal care and pediatric immunizations. The public health system is divided into basic health units (BHUs). Each BHU employs approximately 20 LHWs and a LHW supervisor (LHS). The LHS has a high school education and is hired by the local health department to educate families about pregnancy and infant care with the goal of decreasing infant morbidity and mortality. The LHS leads weekly meetings with the LHWs to discuss issues they are facing with the 200 families in their caseload.

## Building Baby Brains

### BBB curriculum

BBB training attempts to strengthen infant resiliency and support maternal mental health by filling a knowledge gap among LHWs, whose primary training focuses on immunization and nutrition. BBB includes current scientific information about pregnancy, the transition to parenthood, infant development, and a clinical method for strengthening the infant-parent relationship, Thula Sana (Cooper et al., 2009; Valades et al., 2021). Thula Sana is a manualized training for home health visitors derived from the Neonatal Behavioral Assessment Scale (Nugent & Brazelton, 1989). It begins with prenatal visits focusing on the mother's health and on helping her prepare for delivery and the postnatal period. Postnatal visits involve assessing the baby's behavior and interactivity through a series of maneuvers eliciting the infant's strengths and sensitivities, such as demonstrating the infant's motor strength and responsiveness to the caregiver. In revealing to the mother her infant's competencies and behavioral cues, the intervention aims to increase the mother's sensitivity to the baby and strengthen the infant-parent relationship.

The BBB curriculum, both didactic and practical, was developed in the form of training slides, which were then translated into Urdu by native speakers on the research team. The slides were illustrated with photographs of Pakistani infants and caregivers. The pages were printed out and organized into manuals for distribution to the LHWs. In addition to the manual, kits including instruments for the behavioral assessment – pen light, rattle, red ball, and a laminated card with the items for observation – were prepared for the LHWs.

A similar curriculum called "Protect, Nurture, and Enjoy" (PNE) was developed through pilot courses in infant mental health taught to student nurses in North India for five years. Differences between the two curricula included the fact that the PNE curriculum included more biological information, consistent with their nursing training, and the nursing students were not trained to provide a specific clinical intervention.

### Structure of training and supervision

One BHU in South Punjab was identified for the LHWs to receive the BBB training in addition to their standard training. The BBB training was conducted in two-hour session twice per week over four weeks. The training was delivered in the form of remote lectures given by a child psychiatrist in the US (AMH) supported by a Pakistani child psychiatrist practicing in the US, also remote (MZ). An onsite Pakistani pediatrician (SP) also supported the training and provided consecutive translation. The lectures were illustrated by video content and supplemented by a manual provided to each LHW, which contained the lecture content (Appendix).

Following the lectures, SP guided the LHWs in practicing Thula Sana with dolls and demonstrated with a live infant and parent. After completing the BBB training, the LHWs attended two two-hour mentorship meetings of extended practical training. In these meetings, the LHWs worked in pairs to role play the intervention. Following the formal training, the LHWs continued to meet in mentorship groups monthly to discuss their experiences with the implementation of the BBB.

## Approach to outcome study and initial qualitative findings

The outcome study evaluates the effects of the BBB intervention on the care provided to infants and their families by comparing BBB-trained LHWs and the families in their care with a group of LHWs receiving standard training and the families in their care. Two groups will be compared using measures of the LHW knowledge of infant mental health and LHW job satisfaction; maternal psychiatric symptoms; mothers' satisfaction with their care by LHWs and the knowledge they gained from it; and a measure of mother-infant interaction.

### Outcome measures

In order to assess the impact of the BBB training on LHWs, the research team referred to existing health worker knowledge and job satisfaction surveys to develop the LHW Knowledge Survey and the LHW Job Satisfaction Survey (Ahmad et al, 2020, MacPhee, 1981)." The knowledge survey is a 17-item mixed multiple choices and true/false survey covering the content of the BBB training. The job satisfaction survey is a 20-item survey created by the research team to assess the motivation of LHWs to care for families. It was developed from a survey used to explore the motivation of LHWs to engage more actively in tuberculosis case-finding (Khan et al., 2019).

To assess the impact of the intervention on maternal mental health, we used a series of measures that have been validated in perinatal populations to assess depression, anxiety, and trauma. These included the 9-item Patient Health Questionnaire (PHQ-9) (Spitzer et al., 1999), the 7-item Generalized Anxiety Disorder (Spitzer et al., 2006), the PTSD Checklist (Ashbaugh et al., 2016; Blanchard et al., 1996), the Traumatic Events Questionnaire (Crawford et al., 2008), and the Multidimensional Scale of Perceived Social Support (Zimet et al., 1990).

Finally, to assess the impact on mother-infant interaction, we used the Nugent Parent Satisfaction Survey and the Nursing Child Assessment Satellite Training (NCAST) Parent/Child Interaction Scale (Mischenko et al., 2004). The Nugent survey includes questions about the caregiver's understanding of her infant's cues, her self-confidence as a mother, and her satisfaction with her care by the LHW. The NCAST feeding scale was used to assess sensitivity and contingent caregiving in the infant-caregiver relationship at six months. This scale was chosen as a measure because it includes maternal sensitivity items, infant's clarity of cues, and "contingency items" and in that way offers a way of assessing qualities of the relationship and not exclusively of the mother's behavior. Videos of a mother-infant feeding episodes were recorded by LHWs and viewed by a member of the coding team. Each team member completed a training and met the NCAST reliability standard. A portion of the videos were double coded as an additional check on reliability.

These instruments were translated into Urdu and back translated into English by two bilingual members of the study team. The responses to the surveys were also translated into English. Both Urdu and English responses were preserved.

### Stories reported by LHWs

Story from a prenatal visit: A LHW noticed that one of her pregnant I-Ms looked tired and drawn and asked her what was wrong. The mother told her that her husband had announced if she gave birth to a second daughter; he would divorce her and marry a woman who could give him a son. He also spoke harshly to her and sometimes even hit her. At that moment, the husband returned to the house, and the LHW told him that she would like to speak to him privately outside. She explained to him that his baby was listening inside the womb and that the baby heard angry voices. She said that the baby's development could be harmed by the mother's stress. She told him that if he wanted a healthy baby, he would have to treat his wife kindly. She gave him her card. Later, he called her and told her that since their conversation, when he talks to his wife, he speaks as if there were three people in the room. The LHW explained to the group that she had learned about infants listening to outside voices from the womb and about stress being harmful to the fetus, from BBB training.

Story from the one-month visit: During a visit to an intervention group family, the mother left the house to get tea for the LHW, and while she was away, the infant began to cry. When the mother returned, the LHW made a halt-hand gesture and told the mother to stop at the door and speak to the baby. The mother spoke to the baby, and the baby stopped crying. The mother was amazed because she did not know that her voice alone could calm the baby. The grandmother, who entered with the mother, was also amazed. The LHW then told the grandmother to speak to baby, and the baby turned his head to the grandmother's voice. The grandmother was very moved that the baby recognized her voice. The LHW said, "Of course he did. He has been listening from inside the womb, and he said, 'These are my people.'"

## Key points

While this study is still in progress, we would like to highlight a few of the initial findings and remaining questions for future research. First, the BBB training is a powerful intervention. LHWs have reported that the families they serve are interested in learning about infant development and are eager to engage in conversations about the infant-caregiver relationship. Second, most LHWs said that this information was new to them and to the mothers and families in their care, indicating that this type of training is needed. Finally, a family-centered approach appears to be critical to supporting the mother and infant because most of the participating mothers live with their husbands' families and are expected to follow their guidance in matters of childcare. These initial qualitative findings are promising. Once all data have been collected and analyzed, we will know more about the impact of the BBB on LHWs, mothers, and infants. This will allow us to refine the training before expanding to reach a wider population of mothers and infants. It is our goal to support the development of similar programs in Pakistan and other low-resource settings through a process of collaboration with local clinicians and thoughtful adaptation to local culture.

## References

Ahmad, N. F. D., Ren Jye, A. K., Zulkifli, Z., & Bujang, M. A. (2020, Dec). The development and validation of job satisfaction Questionnaire for health workforce. *Malays J Med Sci, 27*(6), 128–143. https://doi.org/10.21315/mjms 2020.27.6.12.

Anda, R. F., Felitti, V. J., Bremner, J. D., Walker, J. D., Whitfield, C., Perry, B. D., Dube, S. R., & Giles, W. H. (2006, Apr). The enduring effects of abuse and related adverse experiences in childhood. A convergence of evidence from neurobiology and epidemiology. *Eur Arch Psychiatry Clin Neurosci, 256*(3), 174–186. https://doi.org/10.1007/s00406-005-0624-4.

Ashbaugh, A. R., Houle-Johnson, S., Herbert, C., El-Hage, W., & Brunet, A. (2016). Psychometric validation of the English and French versions of the posttraumatic stress disorder checklist for DSM-5 (PCL-5). *PLoS One, 11*(10), e0161645. https://doi.org/10.1371/journal.pone.0161645.

Beebe, B., Messinger, D., Bahrick, L., Margolis, A., Buck, K., & Jaffe, J. (2012). Self-regulation is dependent on partner influence, and vice-versa: a dyadic systems view of mother-infant communication. *International Conference Infant Studies*, Minnesota, June 9.

Beeghly, M., Perry, B., & Tronick, E. (2016). Self-regulatory processes in early development. In S. Maltzman (Ed.), *The Oxford handbook of treatment processes and outcomes in psychology: a multidisciplinary, biopsychosocial approach* (pp. 42–54). Oxford University Press. https://doi.org/10.1093/oxfordhb/9780199739134.013.3.

Blanchard, E. B., Jones-Alexander, J., Buckley, T. C., & Forneris, C. A. (1996, Aug). Psychometric properties of the PTSD Checklist (PCL). *Behav Res Ther, 34*(8), 669–673. https://www.ncbi.nlm.nih.gov/pubmed/8870294.

Cooper, P. J., Tomlinson, M., Swartz, L., Landman, M., Molteno, C., Stein, A., McPherson, K., & Murray, L. (2009). Improving quality of mother-infant relationship and infant attachment in socioeconomically deprived community in South Africa: randomised controlled trial. *BMJ, 338*, b974. https://doi.org/10.1136/bmj.b974.

Crawford, E. F., Lang, A. J., & Laffaye, C. (2008, Feb). An evaluation of the psychometric properties of the traumatic events questionnaire in primary care patients. *J Trauma Stress, 21*(1), 109–112. https://doi.org/10.1002/jts.20280.

Felitti, V. J., Anda, R. F., Nordenberg, D., Williamson, D. F., Spitz, A. M., Edwards, V., Koss, M. P., & Marks, J. S. (1998, May). Relationship of childhood abuse and household dysfunction to many of the leading causes of death in adults. The Adverse Childhood Experiences (ACE) Study. *Am J Prev Med, 14*(4), 245–258. https://www.ncbi.nlm.nih.gov/pubmed/9635069.

Fraiberg, S., Shapiro, V., & Adelson, E. (1975). Ghosts in the nursery: a psychoanalytic approach to impaired mother-infant relationships. *JAACAP, 14*(3), 387–421.

Hartmann, H. (1950). Psychoanalysis and developmental psychology. *Psychoanal Study Child, 5*, 7–17. https://doi.org/10.1080/00797308.1950.11822880.

Hughes, K., Bellis, M. A., Hardcastle, K. A., Sethi, D., Butchart, A., Mikton, C., Jones, L., & Dunne, M. P. (2017). The effect of multiple adverse childhood experiences on health: a systematic review and meta-analysis. *Lancet Public Health, 2*(8), e356–e366. https://doi.org/10.1016/s2468-2667(17)30118-4.

Khan, M. S., Mehboob, N., Rahman-Shepherd, A., Naureen, F., Rashid, A., Buzdar, N., & Ishaq, M. (2019, Jul 25). What can motivate Lady Health Workers in Pakistan to engage more actively in tuberculosis case-finding? *BMC Public Health, 19*(1), 999. https://doi.org/10.1186/s12889-019-7326-8.

Lyons-Ruth, K. (1998). Implicit relational knowing: its role in development and psychoanalytic treatment. *Infant Mental Health J, 19*, 282–291.

MacPhee, D. (1981). *Knowledge of infant development inventory manual.* UNC.

Midgley N (2007). Anna Freud: the Hampstead War nurseries and the role of the irect observtion of children for psychoanalysis. *Int J Psychoanal, 4*, 939–959. https://doi.org/10.1516/v28r-j334-6182-524h.

Mischenko, J., Cheater, F., & Street, J. (2004). NCAST: tools to assess caregiver-child interaction. *Community Pract, 77*(2), 57–60.

Monnat, S. M., & Chandler, R. F. (2015, Sep). Long term physical health consequences of adverse childhood experiences. *Sociol Q, 56*(4), 723–752. https://doi.org/10.1111/tsq.12107.

Nugent, J. K., & Brazelton, T. B. (1989). Preventive intervention with infants and families: the NBAS model. *Infant Mental Health J, 10*(2), 84–99. https://doi.org/10.1002/1097-0355(198922)10:2<84::Aid-imhj2280100203>3.0.Co;2-k.

Perry, B. (2019). The Neurosequential Model: a developmentally sensitive, neuroscience-informed approach to clinical problem solving. In J. Tucci, J. Mitchell, & E. Tronick (Eds.), *Evidence-informed approaches to working with traumatized children and adolescents in foster, kinship, and adoptive care* (pp. 137–158). Jessica Kingsley Publishing.

Sander, L. (2014). Living systems, evolving consciousness, and the emerging person: a selection of papers from the life work of Louis Sander, Psychoanalytic Inquiry Book Series, Edited by G. Amadei, & I. Bianchi, v. 26.

Shonkoff, J. P., Garner, A. S., Committee on Psychosocial Aspects of, C., Family, H., Committee on Early Childhood, A., Dependent, C., Section on, D., & Behavioral, P. (2012, Jan). The lifelong effects of early childhood adversity and toxic stress. *Pediatrics, 129*(1), e232–246. https://doi.org/10.1542/peds.2011-2663.

Spitzer, R. L., Kroenke, K., & Williams, J. B. (1999, Nov 10). Validation and utility of a self-report version of PRIME-MD: the PHQ primary care study. Primary Care Evaluation of Mental Disorders. Patient Health Questionnaire. *Jama, 282*(18), 1737–1744. https://www.ncbi.nlm.nih.gov/pubmed/10568646.

Tronick, E. (1989). Emotions and emotional communication in infants. *Am Psychol, 44*(7), 112–119.

Spitzer, R. L., Kroenke, K., Williams, J. B., & Lowe, B. (2006, May 22). A brief measure for assessing generalized anxiety disorder: the GAD-7. *Arch Intern Med, 166*(10), 1092–1097. https://doi.org/10.1001/archinte.166.10.1092.

Sroufe, L. A. (2009, Dec 1). The concept of development in developmental psychopathology. *Child Dev Perspect, 3*(3), 178–183. https://doi.org/10.1111/j.1750-8606.2009.00103.x.

Stern, D. N. (1985). *The interpersonal world of the infant. A view from psychoanalysis and developmental psychology.* Basic Books.

UNICEF. (2021). *UNICEF Data: monitoring the situation of children and women: Pakistan.* https://data.unicef.org/country/pak/.

Valades, J., Murray, L., Bozicevic, L., De Pascalis, L., Barindelli, F., Meglioli, A., & Cooper, P. (2021, May). The impact of a mother-infant intervention on parenting and infant response to challenge: a pilot randomized controlled trial with adolescent mothers in El Salvador. *Infant Ment Health J, 42*(3), 400–412. https://doi.org/10.1002/imhj.21917.

Winnicott, D.W. (1945). Primitive emotional development. *The International Journal of Psychoanalysis, 26,* 137–143.

World Bank. (2019). *Under-five mortality rate.* https://data.worldbank.org/indicator/SH.DYN.MORT?most_recent_value_desc=true.

Zimet, G. D., Powell, S. S., Farley, G. K., Werkman, S., & Berkoff, K. A. (1990, Winter). Psychometric characteristics of the multidimensional scale of perceived social support. *J Pers Assess, 55*(3–4), 610–617. https://doi.org/10.1080/00223891.1990.9674095.

# Part IV
# In search of methods

# 14 The self and self-harm – toward a more nuanced understanding of self-harm in adolescence

*Line Indrevoll Stänicke*

## A historical view on the function of self-harm

Self-harming behavior refers to inflicting pain or injury directly on one's own body, for example by cutting, burning, or hitting oneself. In the general population, 13%–17% of adolescents (12–18 years of age) confirm self-harm (Gillies et al., 2018). In clinical samples, the number is higher; 40%–60% confirm self-harming (Miller et al., 2019). Researchers discuss whether self-harm should include suicidal ideation or not, but regardless of this, the prevalence is approximately the same across different countries.

Importantly, self-harm begins in adolescence, a life period characterized by cognitive, neuro-biological, psychological, and social changes (Thapar et al., 2015). During adolescence, youths develop increased capacity for learning, problem-solving, and abstract thinking, as well as affect regulation and mentalization (Fonagy & Target, 2006), autonomy (Gullestad, 1993), and a more stable self-identity (Erikson, 1968). However, emotional arousal, impulsivity, difficult feelings, and interpersonal stress are often overwhelming, and a need to handle strong feelings is not uncommon. Contact with peers is an important developmental arena for exploring social roles and to learn problem solving. Youths are also more willing to take risks and test boundaries, and risk behavior like drug misuse and self-harm is not uncommon. Today, the digital arenas provided by social media may be understood as an extended peer arena and a possible space for exploring self and others (Stänicke, 2022).

Self-harming behavior raises the question of *why* – why do young people harm themselves? In biblical texts, self-harming was described as instigated by a loss of contact with God (Favazza, 1987). In medical history from the 1800s, examples of serious self-harm – such as the cutting of a limb – and repetitive self-harm – such as "needle picking" – were understood as symptoms of hysteria. Freud (1901) described self-mutilation as motivated by an underlying psychic conflict of sexual drives and later highlighted that self-destructive behavior could be an expression of a compulsion to repeat and a need to process traumatic memories

DOI: 10.4324/9781032651934-19

(Freud, 1914). In addition, he emphasized how self-criticism and self-destructive behavior could be understood as anger directed toward self (Freud, 1917). Some years later, Menninger (1938) proclaimed that self-harm was an expression of self-castration and an unconscious attempt to avoid suicide. He also emphasized that anthropological studies of cultural rituals resembling what we call self-harming praxis were understood as a socially accepted "rite of passage" for group inclusion or a new life stage. In 1969, inspired by Klein and Winnicott and the relational turn in psychoanalysis, Pao (1969) discussed self-harm as a sign of developmental problems in the early emotional relationships. Self-harm was understood as a concrete separation from the mother and as a non-verbal communication exploring the boundaries between an inner and outer world through the body.

Today, several reviews (e.g., Klonsky, 2007; Miller et al., 2019) highlight empirical support for self-harm as having an "affect-regulation" function – the action *regulates* difficult feelings, the person obtains a sense of *control* and achieves something good, a sense of *relief*. Especially, the behavioral perspective underlines how self-harm is reinforced by the increase or decrease of specific inner emotional states or by getting attention or avoiding difficult feelings, thoughts, or difficult situations (Miller et al., 2019). Further, neuro-biological knowledge shows the importance of genetic vulnerability, increased response to stress, and differences in the threshold of pain.

Importantly, case studies and qualitative studies are seldom included in reviews because of lack of statistical power. Further, developmental, socio-cultural, and relational perspectives are rarely represented. In this way, explanations of why people harm themselves are offered at a group level without context-sensitive descriptions. In clinical practice, we know that some cut themselves a few times, others for a temporary period during adolescence, and still others for long periods with serious mental health problems, addiction, low work ability, or early death. Some directly harm their body, while others harm themselves indirectly by engaging in risky behaviors (e.g., driving too fast, or using drugs). In qualitative studies, subjective experience and meaning making can be studied systematically. This knowledge can nuance our understanding of the function of self-harm in adolescence from the youths' perspective. Self-harm may be an overdetermined behavior that serves several functions and needs in different life periods (Soyemoto, 1998).

## A meta-synthesis

A meta-synthesis is a way to analyze and integrate findings from qualitative studies (Levitt et al., 2016). A meta-synthesis of 21 qualitative studies on adolescents' experiences of self-harm, which included a total of more than 500 adolescents 12–18 years of age from different parts of the world, resulted in four meta-themes (Stänicke et al., 2018). First meta-theme, *to obtain release*, is illustrated by this quote:

I don't always cut to make a point, I cut because I need to … when I cut, when I see the blood, and I feel it rushing, it's such relief. I can feel it; it's like everything that is (bad) is just going out.

(Machoian, 2001, p. 26)

Second meta-theme, *to control difficult feelings*, is exemplified in this way: "For once I had a sense of control on my body" (Ayerst, 2005, p. 93). Third meta-theme, *to represent unacceptable feeling*, can be described like this: "I hate anger. I can't do it. When I show it, I try to stop it right away. I harm myself instead" (Holley, 2016, p. 70). Fourth meta-theme, *to connect with others*, is illustrated in this way:

When they see it, like actually see it (a cut), they're like, wow, maybe something is wrong. People won't believe that something is wrong (…) But if they see a cut along a vein, they get the message right away.

(Machoian, 2001, p. 25)

The first two meta-themes bring empirical support for understanding self-harm as affect regulation. Still, self-harm may also be an attempt to communicate – a way to represent and share emotional and relational information without words. Self-harm can be understood as "the voice of the skin" (McLane, 1996), as psychic pain "written on the body" (Adshead, 2010), and "the body becomes a canvas" for mental pain (Lemma, 2010).

Strikingly, many of the quotes from the adolescents in the meta-synthesis underline how self-harm is closely related to a relational context. By using their body, they handle difficult experiences in a self-sufficient manner, keeping their difficulties in a private world and avoid being a burden and *protect* their parents or friends. We discuss whether self-harm may express *a conflict* between attaining autonomy, a developmental challenge in adolescence, and finding one's own ways to handle difficulties on the one hand, *and* a relational need for support and comfort on the other hand (Stänicke et al., 2018).

Learning how to handle problems and overcome difficult feelings may be closely related to sharing one's experiences with others. The relational emotional context is of main importance for developing self-understanding, self-toleration, and a more stable self-identity (Erikson, 1968; Fonagy & Target, 2006; Winnicott, 1971). Thus, self-harm can be understood not only as affect regulation but also as *an attempt* to communicate *in* a relational context. This finding is in line with other authors who underscore that self-harming has an outreaching and sharing function – self-harm is "a cry for help" (Kwawer, 1980), it "cuts the silence" (Brady, 2014), and may bring "a sign of hope" (Motz, 2010).

**Different ways into self-harm – three sub-types**

In my own research on self-harm, I interviewed 21 adolescents, 12–18 years of age, 19 girls, and 2 boys, from a clinical population (Stänicke et al., 2020). We included structured interviews on symptom disorders and personality disorders, and the Adolescent Attachment Interview. For an overview of the results, see Figure 14.1.

All the youths began to harm themselves to handle difficult feelings and relational problems. They often first learned to experiment with self-harm from friends, peers, or self-harm content online. Few of them had close friends, many had an experience of being bullied or isolated socially, feeling that they could not be honest with anybody. In the first interview, at the beginning of their treatment at a public health clinic, they did not see self-harm as a problem or a behavior they needed help with. They were ambivalent toward help, treatment, and ending self-harm, as they had finally found a way to handle problems. Even though they knew their parents were worried and cared for them, they felt unable to turn to them for help, as they did not want to be a burden or make anyone sad or angry. Unfortunately, their attempt to be self-sufficient and hide their problems from others may, in the long run, inhibit and disturb further development of relational reciprocity.

Importantly, despite the similarities among the adolescents' symptoms of self-harm and the common themes of ways into self-harm, there were differences in their descriptions of self-harming episodes – both in semantic content and *how* they represented and integrated affective experiences and their behavior. In the following, these differences are illustrated by three cases – Anna, Elsa, and Sophia – which represent three prototypical sub-types (Stänicke, 2021). The sub-types include differences in self-states during self-harm, in the purpose of self-harm, in self-descriptions, and in the role of others. I argue that these three sub-types show how the concrete cutting is associated with difficult self-experiences that are integrated in different degrees in their self-representation.

*Sub-type 1: The punished self – I deserve it*

Anna began to harm herself when she was 12 years of age. Her parents were in a great conflict, and she felt criticized by her mother about her weight. In addition, a friend had spread rumors about her at school. Anna emphasized that she harmed herself to handle a negative self-image: "I felt disgusting and worthless", she said. The first sub-type represents a *self-state* during self-harm that is dominated by unacceptable and conflicting yet differentiated feelings and thoughts like hate and anger toward herself: "I wanted to give myself pain because I was how I was". The *function* of self-harm was to escape or hide from conflicting feelings: "I can't be a burden". The *self-experience* during self-harm is summarized

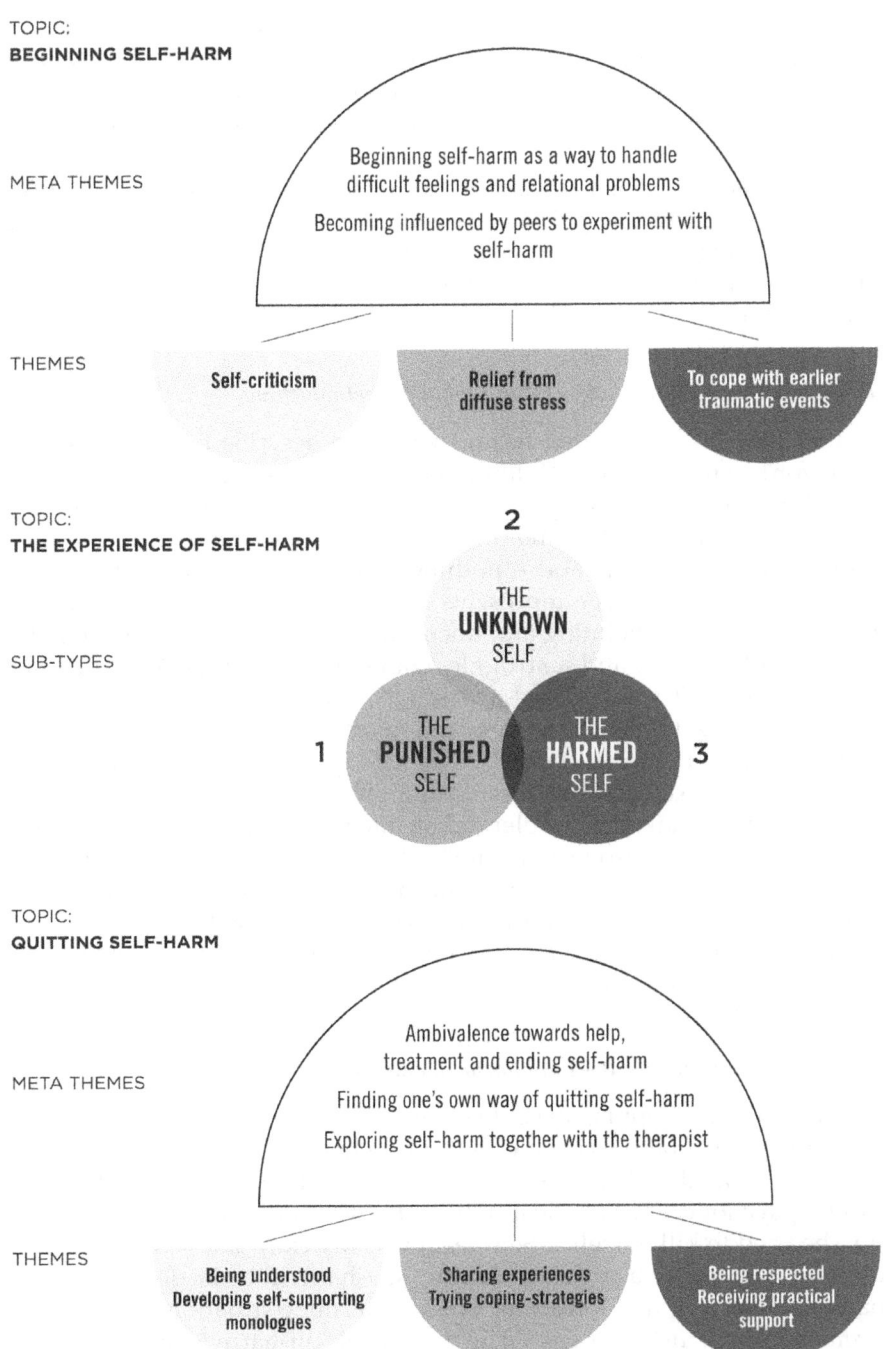

*Figure 14.1* Adolescents' experience of self-harm.

as excessive self-hate: "I deserve pain and punishment for being a bad person". *The role of others* during self-harm may be summarized as an ambivalence about expressing difficult thoughts and feelings toward others. Anna said: "To harm myself (…) is the way I express that I have a difficult time (…) If people don't react, I get sad and think they don't care". She wanted to hide and, at the same time, wanted to be heard. Concretely, self-harm expresses how pain is directed toward the body as punishment instead of being angry, assertive, or defensive toward others. Self-harm may represent frustration with being restricted in life – labeled as "the punished self".

### Sub-type 2: The unknown self – I don't want to feel anything

Another girl, Elsa, struggled to find words to describe her feelings or a reason for harming herself: "I don't really feel very much – in general … I just did it. I don't know why", she said. Despite severe difficulties in her family with somatic and mental illness, Elsa insisted that she had "a nice family and good friends and – nothing traumatic had happened in her life". The second sub-type represents a *self-state* during self-harm that is dominated by overwhelming and uncontrollable anxiety, diffuse feelings, or stressful thoughts, and a struggle against feelings in general, "I can't manage … I don't want to feel anything". The *function* of self-harm becomes a way to get relief from stress and re-establish a sense of control and balance: "I need to feel in control". The *self-experience* during self-harm is summarized as excessively stressful thoughts and feelings that are alien and difficult to understand, tolerate, or integrate as part of oneself. Elsa said: "Something is wrong with me". *The role of others* during self-harm may be described as a perceived need to fulfill others' expectations. Concretely, self-harm may represent how unknown self-experiences are cut off and, at the same time, evoke curiosity and express vulnerability – labeled as "the unknown self".

### Sub-type 3: The harmed self – I am harmed, and no one cares

Yet another girl, Sophia, described self-harming to *overcome traumatic experiences*. Her mother struggled with psychotic illness and had several attempts of suicide: "I was very angry at her as a little girl, but then she got ill – psychotic, she was hospitalized for several periods … Two years ago, she tried to kill herself… Self-harm was my exit," she said. This third sub-type represents a *self-state* during self-harm that is dominated by chaos, being at risk, and left alone. The self-harming situations are difficult to remember: "It just happens". The *function* of self-harm is highlighted as a distraction that makes difficult feelings go away and releases something good: "It is something to rely on". The *self-experience* during self-harm is summarized as being offended, in risk, and that no one cares. *The role of others* during self-harm may be described as a transformation of psychic pain to a physical pain which is easier to share: "It is a way to show I'm hurt". The self-harming act may concretely express the experienced failure of care and, still, represent a way to prevent a psychic breakdown through distraction and re-establish boundaries. The earlier trauma is re-experienced here and now, again and again, through self-harm – labeled as "the harmed self".

### Change – discovering their own way out of self-harm

After one year in treatment, the young people were interviewed again. Most of them had ended self-harming. They especially appreciated their relationship with their therapist, and how the therapist had *explored self-harming episodes* and associated feelings, fantasies, thoughts, actions, and their relational context. Interestingly, the girls did not relate their way out of self-harm to helpful elements in treatment. Rather, they emphasized how *they had found their own way out of self-harm*. Perhaps the experience of discovering their own way can be understood as the girls' attempt to separate and to develop a sense of agency and autonomy. They were, so to speak, "inventing the wheel by themselves".

The three participants described their way out of self-harm differently. Anna emphasized *being understood* by her therapist and how they together explored triggers for self-harming episodes. She developed a *self-supportive monologue*, which served to delay her self-harm:

> I know myself ... this is temporary. The urge goes away. So, I think 'yes, I will harm myself, but first I have to do my homework' (...). Earlier, I only had feelings, and now it's in a way: feelings-stop-think-action. It's wonderful!

For Elsa it was good to *begin talking to someone* about the stress in her life. She developed curiosity about the meaning of these states and discovered how helpful it was to do something else concretely, *trying out new coping strategies*, like the high-intensity exercise of Kick boxing. Most important for Sophie was *to be heard and respected* – just to be allowed to be in the waiting room at the clinic or to get an appointment when she had a hard time. She discovered the possibility of *asking for help*, as well as obtaining medication, care, and support.

> Last week I woke up and just ... fuck life, in a way. It was really bad, and then I called my doctor and asked: 'What should I do?' So, I went and talked to her. She always prioritizes me and gives me the help I need. I have a really good doctor.

Sophie started to accept her vulnerability and dependency. She knew where to get support when needed.

Can these subjective reports increase knowledge of self-harm as a phenomenon? First, we can recognize that the girls' ways into and out of self-harm differ. It is therefore important, especially for therapists, to explore the individual patient's reasons and narrative. Even though we have knowledge about self-harm's "affect-regulating" function – we should not take for granted that we know what it means or what purpose the action has for a particular person. We need to be curious and help patients to explore how self-harm is part of their everyday life.

Second, participants' meaning making may be analyzed in light of the concept of mentalization, defined as a capacity to understand your own and others' behavior in regard of mental content like thoughts, feelings, fantasies, and motives (Fonagy & Target, 2006). Mentalization is operationalized as "reflective functioning" and points to a capacity to represent, integrate, and give meaning to your own and others' experiences and behaviors. The adolescents' ways of describing their subjective reasons for self-harm may indicate different capacity for representing, integrating, and mentalizing important feelings and self-experiences.

Even though Anna had a negative self-focus – hate and anger toward herself – she related self-harming to *parts of herself*. Anna spoke about her problems in a clearly articulated way but tended to internalize problems – she was self-oriented. In difficult situations, Anna perceived her negative thoughts and feelings about herself as the truth and believed everyone else felt the same way about her. Elsa, on the other side, struggled to elaborate and reflect upon what self-harm related to in herself and in her life – it was a *diffuse* form of stress. She *did not want to feel* anything. She had difficulty representing behavior and mental states. We can say that she was non-elaborating or had a non-reflective mode characterized by disavowal, as she was surprised by her own actions. She showed a strong orientation toward others' expectations of her and wanted to be clever at school, the best in sports, the most popular girl, and the best friend. Sophie, who related her self-harming to concrete *dramatic and traumatizing events* and periods in childhood, experienced herself as unpredictable and had problems imagining others' perceptions. She talked about her history in a neutral and non-affective way, but she was still angry at everyone in her everyday life, describing everyone as useless. She tended to externalize problems in general and described self-harm as part of her mental illness. Her anger may have had a protective function.

It also seems plausible that *what* these three participants experienced as helpful in therapy was related to their capacity for mentalization, i.e., exploring difficult situations for Anna, sharing experiences and trying coping strategies for Elsa, and being respected and receiving practical support for Sophie.

### Self-harm – an attempt to represent self

The results of this study highlight how experiences during self-harm seem closely related to youths' experiences and representation of self. Self-punishment as a function of self-harm is emphasized in early psychoanalytic studies (Freud, 1917), and recent studies have underlined self-criticism as common among self-harmers (e.g., Hooley & St Germain, 2014). The action of harming demands energy and determination and the cut can be a channel for expressing power, destructivity, and anger. The concept of *the punished self – I deserve it* (#1) – is suggested as one possible emerging self-representation during self-harming.

Self-harm could also be a way to escape all feelings. Control of difficult feelings is emphasized in the affect-regulation theory (Klonsky, 2007; Miller et al., 2019). Although self-harm seems to have an "affect-regulation" function, a study of the capacity of mentalization highlights the *diversity* among self-harmers. Concretely, self-harm breaks or invades the physical skin – the boundary or protective shield of the inner body from an outer world. The blood that is coming out of an open wound may represent the difficult and alien, and for some, "bad" parts of self. The concept of *the unknown self – I don't want to feel anything* (#2) – highlights how self-harm may be related to one's personal needs.

Self-harm may even prevent a psychic breakdown related to unprocessed trauma of being invaded, forgotten, or assaulted. Several studies emphasize how trauma, sexual or physical abuse, and neglect are risk factors for self-harm (Miller et al., 2019). The motoric action of self-harm may be a possible link between the private and public domain – an attempt to express and communicate unconscious or nonverbal private content through bodily actions to oneself or others (Lemma, 2010; Yakeley & Burbridge-James, 2018). The scars can be signs of inner problems, showing a narrative of their history, a dialogue without words between themselves and their wounds (Gardner, 2001; Straker, 2006). The concept of *the harmed self – I'm harmed, and no one cares* (#3) – underlines how the body can be used to survive psychologically and, at the same time, represents experiences of being neglected.

The three sub-types illustrate how self-experiences are integrated to different degrees – differentiated and conflicting needs (#1), unknown, unrepresented, or diffuse affect (#2), or unprocessed chaotic states related to trauma (#3). These self-experiences are perceived as truths about oneself that must be hidden, controlled, or cut away from self. The results underline the private and individual content that the cut, scars, blood, and wounds invite the person to reflect upon – the need to punish themselves for being angry or bad (#1), the difficulties of expressing and tolerating feelings of vulnerability (#2), or a need for support and care and to process feelings of rejection (#3). Importantly, the youths described loneliness and the fear of bothering their parents or friends with their difficulties. The destructive action of self-harm could be not only an attempt to regulate and to be self-sufficient but also a possibility *to get to know themselves* through the body.

## Some clinical implications

Some structured treatment models show an effect on reducing self-harm, but no treatment models help all patients, and the rates of dropout are high (Hawton et al., 2015). It is still unclear how specific and common treatment factors, and common elements across treatment models, affect the treatment outcome. The three sub-types underline the importance of exploring the *experience* and *function* of self-harm in the patient's everyday life, their *relational context* and *inner world*. In treatment, it is important to focus both on symptom reduction and to understand self-harm as part of self-identity formation. Treatment models may, to different degrees, focus on finding ways to represent and express difficult experiences, on developing alternative coping strategies, or on existential and relational exploration in the therapeutic relationship.

The findings regarding the three sub-types may increase clinicians' ability to understand and explore the developmental challenges of self-identity formation with these vulnerable adolescents *in addition to* affect-regulation problems and processing trauma. If the patient feels understood, self-tolerance and motivation to both end self-harm and explore alternative coping strategies may be enhanced. Further, knowledge of differences in self-representation could involve adjustments to treatment interventions, such as increasing self-reflection and self-compassion (#1), integration of affects (#2), or structural care and practical self-support (#3). Importantly, self-harming girls do not constitute a uniform group.

In a follow-up project, the adolescents were interviewed once again, five years after the first interview (18–25 years of age) (Stänicke, 2022). The focus of the follow-up interview was to explore how they handle difficulties today and whether they have developed alternative ways of coping. For two-thirds of the participants, self-harm was no longer part of their life, and they report struggling less with mental health problems. However, the rest of the participants still harmed themselves occasionally or harmed themselves in more indirect ways, such as drug misuse, risky sex with strangers, being in violent relationships, or eating too little food.

The participants were also invited to explore how self-harm during adolescence was related to digital media engagement and digital risks such as self-harm content online. Even though all participants had extensive social engagement in digital arenas that included self-harm content online, no one shared these experiences with their therapists or other adults during adolescence. They described that despite solitude, engaging in self-harm content online provided them with *a place to fit in*. To look at or share self-harm content online was described as *tempting and a tricky and dangerous game*. One of the participants said: "The bad is good when you are bad". However, they also felt *triggered* when their feed became filled with self-harm content. They felt addicted, afraid of losing their online friends and the online community, and *struggled to end the engagement*. In addition, they felt alone when they dealt with this because *there were no one in charge to help them*.

Interestingly, the participants emphasized how online engagement was like having *an online diary*. Reading about others' problems, sharing their experiences, and learning from others how to handle problems may not only trigger self-harm but also enable self-development by representing difficult, bad, or unknown parts of self. Inspired by Winnicott (1971), we might say that the digital arena has a transitional quality – enabling an intermediate area in between the inner and outer world. For lonely persons, online engagement with self-harm content may enable "a potential space" in between reality and fiction that is sufficient for relational and personal exploration. Engagement in self-harm content online may address a need to belong, to express and share problems, and to obtain support. This knowledge should inform clinicians to ask patients about their engagement in risk content online and to explore how the engagement may be both triggering and helpful in their life.

## References

Adshead, G. (2010). Written on the body: Deliberate self-harm as communication, *Psychoanalytic Psychotherapy*, 24(2), 69–80. doi: 10.1080/02668731003 707501.

Ayerst, S. (2005). *The autobiographical construction of self-harm: A discourse-analytic study of adolescent narratives* (Doctoral dissertation). Available from ProQuest Dissertations and Theses database (UMI No. MR01787).

Brady, M.T. (2014) Cutting the silence: Initial, impulsive self-cutting in adolescence. *International Journal of Child Psychotherapy*, 40, 287–301. doi: 10.1080/0075417X. 2014.965430.

Erikson, E.H. (1968). *Identity: Youth and crisis*. New York: Norton.

Favazza, A.R. (1987). *Bodies under siege. Self-mutilation, nonsuicidal self-injury, and body modification in culture and psychiatry* (3rd ed.). Baltimore, MD: The Johns Hopkins University Press.

Fonagy, P. & Target, M. (2006). The mentalization-focused approach to self-pathology. *Journal of Personality Disorders*, 20, 544–576. doi: 10.1521/pedi.2006. 20.6.544.

Freud, S. (1901). The psychopathology of everyday life. *Standard edition, 6*, 1–239. Translated by J. Strachey. London: Vintage & Hogarth Press.

Freud, S. (1914). Remembering, repeating and working-through (Further recommendations on the technique of psycho-analysis II). *Standard edition, 12*, 146–156. Translated by J. Strachey. London: Vintage & Hogarth Press.

Freud, S. (1917). Mourning and melancholia. *Standard edition*, 14, 239–259. Translated by J. Strachey. London: Vintage & Hogarth Press.

Gardner, F. (2001). *Self-harm. A psychotherapeutic approach*. East Sussex: Brunner-Routledge.

Gillies, D., Christou, M.A., Dixon, A.C., Featherston, O.J., Rapti, I., Garcia-Anguita, A., et al. (2018). Prevalence and characteristics of self-harm in adolescents: Meta-analyses of community-based studies 1990-2015. *Journal of American Academy of Child and Adolescent Psychiatry, 57*(10), 733–741. doi: 10.1016/j.jaac.2018.06.018.

Gullestad, S.E. (1993). A contribution to the psychoanalytic concept of autonomy. *The Scandinavian Psychoanalytic Review, 16*(1), 22–34. doi: 10.1080/01062301. 1993.10592286.

Hawton, K., Witt, K.G., Taylor Salisbury, T.L., Arensman, E., Gunnell, D., Townsend, E., et al. (2015). Interventions for self-harm in children and adolescents. *Cochrane Database of Systematic Reviews, 12,* CD012013. doi: 10.1002/14651858.CD012013.

Holley, E.E. (2016). *The lived experience of adolescents who engage in nonsuicidal self-injury* (Doctoral dissertation). Retrieved from Open Access Theses and Dissertations. (Record No. https://aura.antioch.edu/cgi/viewcontent. cgi?article=1244&context=etds).

Hooley, J.M. & St Germain, S.A. (2014). Nonsuicidal self-injury, pain, and self-criticism: Does changing self-worth change pain endurance in people who engage in self-injury? *Clinical Psychology Science, 2*(3), 297–305. doi: 10.1177/ 2167702613509372.

Klonsky, E.D. (2007). The functions of deliberate self-injury: A review of the evidence. *Clinical Psychology Review, 27,* 226–239. doi: 10.1016/j.cpr.2006.08.002.

Kwawer, J.S. (1980). Some interpersonal aspects of self-mutilation in a borderline patient. *Journal of American Academy of Psychoanalysis, 8*(2), 203–216. PMID: 7358536.

Lemma, A. (2010). *Under the skin. A psychoanalytic study of body modification*. London: Routledge.

Levitt, H.M., Pomerville, A., & Surace, F. (2016). A qualitative meta-analysis examining clients' experiences of psychotherapy: A new agenda. Psychological Bulletin, *142*(8), 801–830. doi: 10.1037/bul0000057.

Machoian, L. (2001). Cutting voices. *Journal of Psychosocial Nursing & Mental Health Services, 39*(11), 22–29.

McLane, J. (1996). The voice on the skin: Self-mutilation and Merleau-Ponty's theory of language. *Hypatia, 11,* 107–118. doi: 10.1111/j.1527-2001.1996.tb01038.x.

Menninger, K. (1938/1966). *Man against himself*. New York: Brace World Inc.

Miller, A.B., Massing-Schaffer, M., Owens, S., & Prinstein, M.J. (2019). Nonsuicidal self-injury among youth. In T.H. Ollendick, S.W. White, & B.A. White (Eds.), *The Oxford handbook of clinical child and adolescent psychology*. Oxford: Oxford University Press. doi: 10.1093/oxfordhb/9780190634841.013.34.

Motz, A. (2010). Self-harm as a sign of hope. *Psychoanalytic Psychotherapy, 24,* 81–92. doi: 10.1080/02668731003707527.

Pao, P.-N. (1969). The syndrome of delicate self-cutting. *British Journal of Medical Psychology, 42,* 195–206. doi: 10.1111/j.2044-8341.1969.tb02071.x.

Soyemoto, K.L. (1998). The functions of self-mutilation. *Clinical Psychology Review, 18,* 531–554. doi: 10.1016/S0272-7358(97)00105-0.

Stänicke, L.I., Haavind, H., & Gullestad, S.E. (2018). How do young people understand their own self-harm? A meta-synthesis of adolescents' subjective experience of self-harm. *Adolescent Research Review, 3,* 173–191. doi:10.1007/ s40894-018-0080-9.

Stänicke, L.I., Haavind, H., Rø, F.G., & Gullestad, S.E. (2020). Discovering one's own way: Adolescent girls' different pathways into and out of self-harm. *Journal of Adolescent Research, 35*(5), 605–634. doi:10.1177/0743558419883360.

Stänicke, L.I. (2021). The punished self, the unknown self, and the harmed self – Toward a more nuanced understanding of self-harm among adolescents. *Frontiers of Psychology*, *12*, 543303. doi: 10.3389/fpsyg.2021.543303.

Stänicke, L.I. (2022). "I chose the bad" – Youth's meaning making of being involved in self-harm content online during adolescence. *Child & Family Social Work*, *28*(1), 160–170.

Straker, G. (2006). Signing with a scar: Understanding self-harm. *Psychoanalytic Dialogues*, *16*, 93–112. doi: 10.2513/s10481885pd1601_6.

Thapar, A., Pine, D.S., Leckman, J.F., Scott, S., Snowling, M.J., & Taylor, E. (2015). *Child and adolescent psychology* (6h ed.). West Sussex: John Wiley and Sons, Ltd.

Winnicott, D.W. (1971). *Playing and reality*. London: Routledge.

Yakeley, J. & Burbridge-James, W. (2018). Psychodynamic approaches to suicide and self-harm. *The British Journal of Psychiatry Advances*, *24*, 37–45. doi: 10.1192/bja.2017.6.

# 15 Relational competence in psychotherapy

*Cecilie Hillestad Hoff*

## Introduction

One of the most robust empirical findings of psychotherapy research in recent years is that therapists differ in their average effectiveness. A recent review concludes that these so-called therapist effects have been found consistently across different clinical settings and patient groups and are estimated to account for approximately 5% of the variance in outcome measures (Johns et al., 2019). In contrast to this consistent support for the relevance of therapist effects, it is less clear which therapist characteristics are responsible for these effects (Heinonen & Nissen-Lie, 2019). One therapist variable of interest is therapists' relational skills (Munder et al., 2019). However, as Hill et al. (2017) emphasize, after decades of research, the question of how relational skills should be operationalized still represents a knowledge gap in the field. As such, it seems urgent to understand more about the nature of good therapeutic skills, and how they are achieved.

In this chapter, I will examine the nature of *relational therapeutic competence*. I will use this as a concept including interpersonal skills, emotional skills, and a capacity to detect, contain, and use one's countertransference feelings. In the research literature, however, the concept *relational skills* is a more commonly used term, referring more specifically to therapists' observable behavior. As such, when referring to studies investigating this, I will use the term *relational skills*.

As the performance of relational skills always takes place within the context of a human, complex, and individualized process, it is difficult to empirically investigate and come to any definite answers about these processes and their associated outcomes (Knox & Hill, 2021). Nevertheless, there is enthusiasm within the research field about developing new methods that may contribute to shedding light on the nature of relational competence and skills. I will explore some of these developments and particularly focus on how therapists must play on different knowledge modalities, including both verbal and nonverbal aspects.

Moreover, I will argue that the recent developments within the psychotherapy research area, with its focus on the significance of the patient-therapist

DOI: 10.4324/9781032651934-20

relationship, can bring psychoanalysis closer to academic psychology and the psychotherapy research field. Also, I will emphasize how psychoanalytic researchers, by following the principles of inductive qualitative research methods, can increase the scientific quality of psychoanalytic research. Finally, I will give a brief presentation of an ongoing study demonstrating how psychoanalytic qualitative research can produce useful knowledge both about relational competence, and the more specific skills that are part of this competence, that convincingly explains phenomena that are difficult to understand from a cognitive or rational perspective. I will start this chapter by giving a brief introduction to qualitative research and explore some of its inherent challenges.

## Qualitative research

As Corbin and Strauss (2015) underline, qualitative data analysis is both an art and a science. The creative aspect of the analytic process "requires knowing what ideas to pursue, how far to develop an idea, when to let go, and how to keep a balance between conceptualization and description" (ibid., p. 65). The researcher must remain flexible and creative in the way procedures are used to solve analytic problems, be able to think outside the box, and be willing to take risks. The science aspect of qualitative research is anchored in the way interpretations are grounded in the data. In qualitative analysis, interpretations are not wild guesses or based on intuition, but a result of a systematic and time-consuming analytic process, where the researcher's understanding of the data is always validated against further data (Blumer, 1969).

Qualitative research has a distinctive strength in its potential to be *enriching*. It seeks to deepen people's understanding of a phenomenon by considering it from different perspectives, uncovering the implicit and explicit meanings involved (Levitt et al., 2021). Hence, this form of research can capture nuances and details in the research material that may be overlooked by a research design that in many contexts is regarded as a gold standard, like randomized controlled trials (RCTs). An RCT design relies on a battery of widely used and validated outcome measures, including structured interviews and self-reported questionnaires. This makes it possible to have confidence in the reliability and validity of the measures and to compare findings across a range of different studies. However, it also means that the only outcomes being measured are the ones that have been predetermined by the researchers. These predetermined measures are, of course, influenced by existing theories, concepts, and ideas. The qualitative research process, on the other hand, is a more dynamic process where the research questions and hypotheses are constantly evaluated and altered, informed by the research process. As such, an advantage with qualitative research is that it can produce knowledge that is unexpected and surprising, thus challenging existing theories and ideas.

One of the most central challenges related to qualitative research is concerned with *generalizability*. A common critique is that research results from qualitative studies, due to small data samples, cannot be generalized (Roald et al., 2021). However, as Osbeck and Antczak (2021) underline, generalizations in qualitative research do not aim to extend findings to whole populations but rather try to capture the lived phenomenon in all its dimensionality. This means that generalizations are not extracted from a sample of participants, but from a set of observations. Thus, qualitative research aims to understand the meaning in a phenomenon, not simply to assess the number of people featuring one characteristic or whether specific variables are present or not. In this perspective, qualitative research is not based upon small sample sizes but can be considered to generate an endless number of possible observations and analyses (Levitt, 2021).

When studying relational competence, researchers would not simply look for the presence, or absence, of such competence, but rather explore variances in the therapeutic interventions and how these affect the patient. Moreover, it is important to incorporate how the patient and the therapeutic relationship influence the therapist, to convey whether there is something in the relational dynamic that may put the therapist's relational competence to the test. When patterned meanings across such themes occur in the data material, it is possible to develop an understanding that may have a validity that is germane beyond this material.

Two qualitative approaches that have been increasingly used as methodological frameworks within qualitative psychological research during the last decades are interpretative phenomenological analysis (IPA) and reflexive thematic analysis (RTA). They both represent an *idiographic* perspective; that is, they aim to reveal something about the particular. Hence, they usually study small samples and produce detailed and nuanced knowledge which we cannot obtain through experimental studies and large sample research designs (Flyvbjerg, 2006; Smith et al., 2009). The term *reflexive* refers to how researchers during a research process must demonstrate a critical reflection on the research, both as process and as practice. This requires that researchers reflect on their own theoretical positions, and how these shape and influence production of knowledge (Braun & Clark, 2013).

Moreover, IPA and RTA are both concerned with how researchers must meet their raw data with openness and reflexivity. Thus, they emphasize how qualitative research must follow the principles of a so-called bottom-up perspective. Using raw data as a vantage point, the researcher during the analytic process develops *themes* that in turn give patterned meaning across a dataset that captures something essential about the data in relation to the research question (Braun & Clark, 2006, 2019). Later in the research process, theoretical reflections are brought in to develop theories that can explain these patterned meanings. Hence, new knowledge may strengthen existent theories, or contradict previous findings, and thus contribute to challenge existing theories and beliefs.

### Relational skills

The robust empirical foundation for the existence of *therapist effects*, referring to "the conjecture that some therapists achieve better therapy outcomes with their patients than do other therapists" (Wampold & Owen, 2021, p. 300), has turned our focus toward the person of the therapist. Still, as Castonguay and Hill (2017) highlight, therapist effects represent an intriguing paradox within psychotherapy research. Although we intuitively know that therapists differ in their effectiveness, the empirical evidence that explains these differences is still scarce. Empirical studies investigating whether different therapist characteristics such as therapists' attachment style, gender, and level of experience are related to outcome measures have so far produced contradictory findings (Wampold & Owen, 2021).

However, a growing amount of empirical evidence indicates that interpersonal skills in emotionally challenging contexts are a core feature of effective therapists (Wampold & Owen, 2021). A recent line of studies has focused on what the researchers call facilitative interpersonal skills (FIS), measured by the therapist's ability to capture the interpersonal style of the client, and respond in ways that challenge this pattern (Anderson et al., 2009, 2015, 2016a, 2016b, 2020). This research paradigm makes use of an experimental design, where actors are instructed to enact short sequences of specific challenging relational scenarios. These brief sections are video recorded and then showed individually to groups of psychotherapists, who are asked to respond as they would have done in real therapy. The participants' responses are then coded for eight skills: verbal fluency, emotional expressiveness, warmth/understanding, empathy, persuasiveness, hope, alliance-bond capacity, and rupture-repair responsiveness. Each therapist's FIS score is later analyzed in relation to outcomes in real therapy processes. These studies have been replicated several times and have consistently lent credence to the view that therapists' FIS score is an independent contributor to therapeutic alliance and outcome.

By demonstrating that it is possible to operationalize and measure relational skills, the FIS paradigm represents a considerable contribution to the research fields. However, due to the experimental design, these studies do not shed light on how relational skills develop over time in real therapy settings. Moreover, the outcome measures are based on short therapy processes, and therefore, they do not tell us anything about mechanisms involved in more intensive processes over time. Finally, therapists in these studies are responding to actors acting like patients on a video screen. It seems reasonable to question in what sense these relational sequences can capture the dynamic complexities inherent in therapeutic relationships. All in all, then, we need more knowledge of how to understand FIS, and how they should be applied with different patients and in different contexts (Wampold & Flückiger, 2022).

## From observation to theory

An increasing number of investigators today aim at uncovering *how* therapeutic change happens (Pascual-Leone & Greenberg, 2007). Hence, there is a request within the field for systematic qualitative studies investigating psychotherapeutic processes and mechanisms. By describing the structure of therapeutic processes from a stance close to experience, researchers aim to capture what therapists actually do in naturalist therapy settings, rather than what they say they do. This perspective takes into consideration how subtle or implicit interactions and enactments may influence the clinical situation over time. Whereas the FIS studies primarily investigate the performative aspects of relational skills, naturalistic studies based on observation can generate more nuanced knowledge capturing a wider specter of relational competence.

In line with the principles of IPA and RTA described earlier, Schachter and Kächele (2017) argue that this focus on the immediacy of the therapeutic encounter is not compatible with top-down research strategies but requires a methodological shift toward bottom-up research. Hence, researchers should avoid looking for how clinical examples can illustrate theory but rather try to convey how observations of naturalistic therapy processes can highlight and help us break down the concept *relational competence,* to develop a meaningful and clinically relevant operationalization of the different skills involved.

As psychoanalysis is a strong theoretical discipline, some may argue that it is particularly challenging for researchers from a psychoanalytic perspective to conduct sound qualitative bottom-up research. At its worst, psychoanalytic research is theory driven, using a case study or a clinical example to demonstrate a theoretical concept. At its best, psychoanalytic research is conducted as a process close to an observational stance, using these observations as a vantage point for developing theoretical explanations. Such an observational stance is deeply rooted in the psychoanalytic project. Freud wrote: "For these ideas are not the foundation of the science upon which everything rests. That foundation is observation alone" (1914, p. 77). For psychoanalysis to be in a fruitful dialogue with academic psychology, it needs to cultivate this observational stance and conduct research in line with principles of bottom-up research.

Researchers from different theoretical positions are now increasingly using direct observations of naturalistic therapy sessions for investigating psychotherapeutic processes and mechanisms behind change (Altimir & Jiménéz, 2021). Several studies have accentuated how therapists must attend to a continuous stream of information from patients, communicated through both verbal and nonverbal channels, such as gaze behavior, facial expressions, and body posture (Bennecke et al., 2005). In this perspective, the therapeutic encounter is a fundamentally multi-channel process. Verbally, both therapists and clients can express intentions to explore emotional topics.

At the same time, nonverbal cues, such as averted eye gaze or body lean-ing away, may signal difficulties in exploring these emotions. To promote change, then, therapists must be able to play on different knowledge mo-dalities to inform their clinical understanding and interventions (Oddli & McLeod, 2017).

In an ongoing single case study based on careful and systematic analy-sis of video recordings of a psychodynamic psychotherapy training and supervision process, we aim at investigating how the therapist integrates verbal and nonverbal knowledge modalities.[1] It is beyond the scope of this chapter to go into depth about methodology and findings. The intention here is to demonstrate how a qualitative, bottom-up study of the develop-ment of relational competence can work as a starting point from where psy-choanalytic theory can contribute with relevant perspectives to interpret the data results.

In line with the principles of RTA, we started the research process with open observations of the video-recorded material. Later, two interviews were conducted with the student therapist and the patient, respectively. We also collected an independent reflection note from the clinical super-visor in the case, where she was asked to focus on her understanding of the process in general, and the development of the therapist, the patient, and the therapeutic relationship. The research group consists of four re-searchers, where three are anchored in a psychoanalytic perspective and one in an integrative perspective. During the first phase of the research process, when observing the video-recorded material, we openly discussed our theoretical positions and focused on trying to meet the data material open-mindedly, constantly with an awareness of potential theoretical pre-conceptions. As such, we had to increase our awareness of implicit as well as explicit theoretical perspectives of the topic under study and be willing to put them under scrutiny.

During our initial observations, we were drawn to the nonverbal com-munication within the therapeutic dyad, which was recognized by a lot of tension, both in the therapist and in the client. Hence, informed by the research process, our research question gradually moved toward nonver-bal expressions and interactions. Close observations of the video-recorded material revealed that the therapist's body language expressed a sense of insecurity which caught our attention. For example, she could sit down in the beginning of a session with a deep sigh, smile, or giggle inappropri-ately, pick on her clothes or fiddle with her key card, comb through her hair with her fingers several times or collect her hair over one shoulder. The patient also showed some typical nonverbal behavioral patterns which made him look insecure and uncomfortable. He would typically smile a lot during sessions, not because they shared a sense of joy or had made a humoristic remark. Rather, he would often smile in situations where there was a silence in the room, and where he expressed that he did not know what to say. He would also typically sit with his legs crossed, swinging the one on top in a repetitive manner, take his wristwatch on and off several times during a session, and withdrawing his gaze, looking down on the floor or looking around at the room.

Video recordings of the supervision sessions revealed that the therapist during supervision had a different nonverbal behavioral pattern than during therapy sessions. In supervision, she was calm and natural. She came forward as competent and skilled, and she was able to reflect on the therapeutic relationship and her own role as a therapist. Moreover, during the interviews, neither the therapist nor the patient showed any signs of nonverbal insecurity. Hence, there was reason to believe that there was something in the therapeutic relationship that created a nonverbal tension. In our further analysis, we were trying to explore and understand these paradoxical behavior patterns.

In the beginning of the first interview, both the therapist and the patient, without being told that nonverbal communication was the topic of the study, were asked about their immediate thoughts about the process. They both, independently, commented on their body language and the nonverbal interactions in the sessions. For example, the therapist said that what first came to her mind was how the patient in the first part of the process seemed ill at ease nonverbally and noted that he became calmer toward the end of the process. She also expressed that her patient's body language made her feel insecure, and that she remembered feeling a tension between them. She experienced this tension as an expression of her patient's difficulties using the therapy to come forward with his feelings. Moreover, she emphasized that she had a strong sense that the patient wanted her to take the lead during sessions, and how she had to work very hard to make him take the lead and allow himself to be more autonomous in the relationship and his life outside the therapy setting. The patient, in his interview, also commented on his own bodily uneasiness, stating that he remembered "being all over the place". Later, when asked about his thoughts on his own nonverbal behavioral pattern, he revealed that he thought it was an expression of insecurity and the discomfort he felt being in the room with the therapist.

In her description note, the supervisor, in line with the therapist's reflections during her interview, revealed that there was a struggle in the therapeutic relationship about who was to take the lead during sessions, and that she believed this made the therapist insecure. Her observations were substantiated by the observations of the research team, where we understood the therapist's nonverbal behavior as a response to her patient's underlying anxiety. For example, the therapist's way of smiling or giggling when the patient had difficulties knowing what to say or getting in touch with his underlying emotions was interpreted as a countertransference reaction, where she was "infected" by her patient's defensiveness – a specific psychoanalytic perspective. Moreover, as the therapist became particularly insecure and uncomfortable in situations where the patient had difficulties knowing what to say, we theorized that her bodily insecurity could be understood as an expression of a deeper anxiety that was played out in the transference.

According to Sandler's theory of role responsiveness, unconscious fantasies involve internalizations of previous role relationships, in which both self and other objects are represented in particular roles (Sandler, 1976). In the transference, patients may attempt to actualize those role relationships, by unconsciously inviting the analyst to repeat these familiar scenarios. This notion of role responsiveness may shed light on the specific relational dynamics that were played out in our case. We were discussing whether the patient's difficulties with knowing what to say could be an expression of a defense strategy, where he was unconsciously inviting the therapist into taking the lead during sessions. This again was understood as a deeper expression of an anxiety related to come forward with his emotions and thoughts. This interpretation was substantiated by the fact that, during the therapy process, it became clear that the patient repetitively came into situations with his girlfriend where she was the one in charge, and he had to obey her demands, something which caused a lot of frustration and conflict between them.

This brief extract from our study illustrates how an idiographic perspective, as described in the method section, can uncover nuances and complexities that may be missed when investigating larger data samples (Flyvbjerg, 2006). Moreover, bearing in mind how affect is expressed nonverbally within every therapeutic dyad, and how this study can work as a vantage point for discussing internal variances of this topic, it seems reasonable to argue that the issues we discuss may be found relevant and valuable beyond our particular case (Levitt et al., 2021). Finally, our study illustrates how psychoanalytic thinking can help us understand complex, and unconscious, relational interactions that are observed in a data material and thus make it possible for researchers and clinicians from other perspectives to relate to and evaluate psychoanalytic theory. Hence, this form of research can represent a contribution to the academic psychotherapy research area and at the same time to cultivate and strengthen the psychoanalytic clinical and scientific endeavor.

## Note

1 The presentation of the study is approved by the informants.

## References

Altimir, C., & Jiménez, J.P. (2021). The clinical relevance of interdisciplinary research on affect regulation in the analytic relationship. *Frontiers in Psychology*, 12, 718490–718490.

Anderson, T., Ogles. B. M., Patterson, C. L., Lambert, M. J., & Vermeersch, D. A. (2009). Therapist effects: Facilitative interpersonal skills as a predictor of therapist success. *Journal of Clinical Psychology*, 65 (7), 755–768.

Anderson, T., Crowley, M. E. J., Himawan, L., Holmberg, J. K., & Uhlin, B. D. (2015). Therapist facilitative interpersonal skills and training status: A randomized clinical trial on alliance and outcome. *Psychotherapy Research*. http://doi.org/10.1080/10503307.2015.1049671.

Anderson, T., McClintock, A. S., Himawan, L., Song, X., & Patterson, C. L. (2016a). A prospective study of therapist facilitative interpersonal skills as a predictor of treatment outcome. *Journal of Consulting and Clinical Psychology*, 84 (1), 57–66.

Anderson, T., Crowley, M. E. J., Himawan, L., Holmberg, J. K., & Uhlin, B. D. (2016b). Therapists' facilitative interpersonal skills and training status: A randomized clinical trial on alliance and outcome. *Psychotherapy Research*, 26 (5), 511–529.

Anderson, T., Perlman, M. R., McCarrick, S. M., & McClintock, A. S. (2020). Modeling therapist responses with structured practice enhances facilitative interpersonal skills. *Journal of Clinical Psychology*, 76(4), 659–675. https://doi.org/10.1002/jclp.22911.

Bennecke, C., Peham, D., & Bänninger-Huber, E. (2005). Nonverbal relationship regulation in psychotherapy. *Psychotherapy Research*, 15 (1–2), 81–90. https://doi.org/10.1080/10503300512331327065.

Blumer, H. (1969). *Symbolic interactionism: Perspective and method*. Berkeley: University of California Press.

Braun, V., & Clarke. V. (2006). Using thematic analysis in psychology. *Qualitative Research in Psychology*, 3 (2), 77–101. https://doi.org//10.1191/1478088706qp063oa.

Braun, V., & Clarke, V. (2013). *Successful qualitative research. A practical guide for beginners*. London: Sage Publications Ltd.

Braun, V., & Clarke, V. (2019). Reflecting on reflexive thematic analysis. *Qualitative Research in Sport, Exercise and Health*, 11 (4), 589–597. https://doi.org/10.1080/2159676X.2019.1628806.

Castonguay, L. G., & Hill, E. (eds.) (2017). *How and why are some therapists better than others? Understanding therapist effects*. Washington, DC: American Psychological Association.

Corbin, J., & Strauss, A. (2015). *Basics of qualitative research. Techniques and procedures for developing grounded theory*. Thousand Oaks, CA: Sage Publications Inc.

Flyvbjerg, B. (2006). Five misunderstandings about case-study research. *Qualitative Inquiry*, 12 (2), 219–245.

Freud, S. (1914). On narcissism: An introduction. SE 14, 67–102.

Heinonen, E., & Nissen-Lie, H. (2019). The professional and personal characteristics of effective psychotherapists: A systematic review. *Psychotherapy Research*, 30 (4), 417–432.

Hill, C. E., Spiegel, S. B., Hoffman, M. A., Kivlighan, D. M. Jr., & Gelso, C. J. (2017). Therapist expertise in psychotherapy revisited. *The Counseling Psychologist*, 45 (1), 7–53.

Johns, R. G., Barkham, M., Kellett, S., & Saxon, D. (2019). A systematic review of therapist effects: A critical update and refinement to Baldwin and Imel's (2013) review. *Clinical Psychology Review*, 67, 78–93.

Knox, S., & Hill, C. E. (2021). Training and supervision in psychotherapy: What we know and where we need to go. In M. Barkham, W. Lutz, & L. G. Castonguay (eds.), *Bergin and Garfield's handbook of psychotherapy and behavior change* (7th ed., pp. 327–349). New Jersey: John Wiley & Sons.

Levitt, H. (2021). Qualitative generalizations, not to the populations, but to the phenomenon: Reconceptualizing variation in qualitative research. *Qualitative Psychology*, 8(1), 95–110.

Levitt, H., McLeod, J., & Stiles, W. B. (2021). The conceptualization, design, and evaluation of qualitative methods in research on psychotherapy. In M. Barkham, W. Lutz, & L. G. Castonguay (eds.), *Bergin and Garfield's handbook of psychotherapy and behavior change* (7th ed., pp. 51–85). New Jersey: John Wiley & Sons.

Munder, T., Schlipfenbacher, C., Toussant, K., Warmuth, M, Anderson, T., & Gumz, A. (2019). Facilitative interpersonal skills performance test: Psychometric analysis of a German language version. *Journal of Clinical Psychology*, 75, 2273–2283.

Oddli, H. W., & McLeod, J. (2017). Knowing – in – Relation: How experienced therapists integrate different sources of knowledge in actual clinical practice. *Journal of Psychotherapy Integration*, 27, 107–116.

Osbeck, L. M., & Antczak, S. L. (2021). Generalizability and qualitative research: A new look at an ongoing controversy. *Qualitative Psychology*, 8(1), 62–68.

Pascual-Leone, A., & Greenberg, L. S. (2007). Emotional processing in experiential psychotherapy: Why "the only way out is through". *Journal of Consulting and Clinical Psychology*, 75 (6), 875–887.

Roald, T., Køppe. S., Jensen, T. B., Hansen, J. M., & Levin, K. (2021). Why do we always generalize in qualitative research? *Qualitative Psychology*, 8 (1), 69–81.

Sandler, J. (1976). Countertransference and role-responsiveness. *International Review of Psycho-Analysis*, 3 (1), 43–47.

Schachter, J., & Kächele, H. (2017). *Nodal points: Critical issues in contemporary psychoanalytic theory*. New York: IPBoks.

Smith, J. A., Flowers, P., & Larkin, M. (2009). *Interpretative phenomenological analysis. Theory, method, and research*. London: Sage Publications Ltd.

Wampold, B. E., & Owen, J. (2021). Therapist effects: History, methods, magnitude, and characteristics of effective therapists. In M. Barkham, W. Lutz, & L. G. Castonguay (eds.), *Bergin and Garfield's handbook of psychotherapy and behavior change* (7th ed. pp. 297–326). New Jersey: John Wiley & Sons.

Wampold, B. E., & Flückiger, C. (2022). The alliance in mental health care: conceptualization, evidence, and clinical applications. *World Psychiatry*, 22, 25–41.

# 16 Developing therapeutic competence

## Learning to work in the transference

*Hanne Strømme and Stephan Hau*

How do we learn working in the transference? This is a main challenge for becoming a psychoanalyst and a psychodynamic therapist (e.g., Killingmo et al., 2014; Tuckett, 2005). The work involves both an ability to empathize with the evoked feelings of the patient toward oneself in the here-and-now in the therapeutic interaction, to be aware of evoked feelings in oneself, and to act upon this complex understanding to promote the therapeutic process and structural changes in the patient (Gullestad & Killingmo, 2020). A successful learning process will result in various kinds of intrapsychic changes in the trainee (e.g., Fleming & Benedek, 1966; Killingmo et al., 2014).

In this chapter, we will present empirical studies investigating aspects of the learning process necessary for dealing with transference phenomena, discuss the limitations of these studies, and pinpoint needs for further empirical research. Our specific aim is to identify possible intrapsychic changes in the trainees, such as changes in defense reactions and higher tolerance for specific affects and emotions. Moreover, we present an ongoing study within the Nordic Psychotherapy Training Study (NORTRAS) with the purpose of meeting some of these needs.

## Empirical studies of therapist change while learning transference work

The publications we found in a systematic literature search of therapists' learning to work in the transference can be divided into studies of outcome and process. None of the training studies especially highlight learning to work in the transference but rather address psychoanalytic (and psychodynamic) competence in general. Therefore, in the included quantitative studies, we have tried to isolate competence criteria related to transference work and in qualitative research to the researchers' interpretations of transference phenomena.[1]

## Search procedures

Databases PsycINFO and PEP Web (in March 2023) were searched by using terms addressing empirical research (e.g., stud*, surve*, quantitative*),

DOI: 10.4324/9781032651934-21

training (e.g., train*), therapy tradition (e.g., psychodyn*), supervision (e.g., superv*), and transference phenomena (e.g., transferenc*) in various combinations. Inclusion criteria: Trainees (and their patients) and/or supervisors in the psychodynamic tradition; training studies related to working with transferences phenomena; the therapy and supervision couples; research designs. Exclusion criteria: Group processes in group therapy and/or group supervision; studies of transference phenomena within other traditions.

*Training outcome*

A survey study of psychoanalytically oriented training (Buckley et al. 1982) showed increased "Ability to deal with the patients' resistance" and "Ability to understand defensive structures" – based on supervisors' pre- and post-ratings of 29 competency items. However, the three items "Ability to empathize with patients", "To monitor own countertransferences", and "Ability to establish an effective therapeutic alliance" did not receive better scores at the end. The researchers assumed that these skills were related to the personality of the therapist, not easily changed within eight-month training.

The Vanderbilt II study (Henry et al., 1993) investigated changes in therapist behaviors during one year of manual-based training in time-limited dynamic psychotherapy. The therapists acquired more technical skills, which is in line with the results of Hilsenroth et al. (2006), but did not prove the expected advantage of manual-based training. Afterward, the trainees tended to appear less warm and supportive and more authoritarian and defensive, an unexpected deterioration. The authors speculate that trainees may have felt less free to follow their intuitive relational skills, which, we might add, is so important in transference work. Of particular interest, the study also documents the difficulty of handling hostile transferences.

In a pilot study, Ravitz et al. (2019) investigated training outcomes in psychodynamic therapy and cognitive therapy. In psychodynamic training, the residents increased their attendance to emotional arousal in patients and ability to link patients' feelings or perceptions to past situations or behaviors, both fundamental aspects of transference work. The researchers speculated that psychodynamic therapy is more difficult to learn than cognitive therapy. As in the Vanderbilt II study, it was emphasized that adherence is not enough to establish competence, as the interpersonal skills of the therapists determine how the patients perceive and make use of the skills.

In a longitudinal survey and interview study of doctoral students and their clients, the trainees reported improvements in psychodynamic/interpersonal competence during one-year external practice (Hill et al., 2015). The trainees were able to form stronger working alliances and real relationships and were better in facilitating improvement in clients' interpersonal relationships, also rated by their clients. Of relevance here, the trainees stated improvements in countertransference management.

In a study of Killingmo et al. (2014), learning to deal with the transference among pre-graduate psychologists was part of the operationalization of a new concept, "strategic thinking", which refers to "the ability of the therapist to continuously reflect on therapeutic aims and on means designed to achieve these aims", possible for others to observe. The evaluators listened to the fifth last therapy session and described the competence of the trainees in a short essay. Four types of dialogue patterns emerged: (1) strategic thinking, (2) partial strategic thinking, (3) absence of strategic thinking, and (4) anti-therapeutic relations. In the first group, therapists displayed basic dynamic competence, such as letting the patients express themselves at their own pace, were geared to the subjective experience and current feeling state of the patients, and did not seem controlled by a pressing desire to "help" or to "do" something. Moreover, maintaining a respectful and benevolent attitude, they did not take a judgmental position regarding the behavior, feelings, and fantasies of the patients. However, only very few of the trainees in this most competent group were able to formulate interventions based of the understanding of the emotional subtext, that is to work in the transference.

In the second group, the strategic thinking could be lost in periods, and in the third, absent altogether. Here, the student therapists relied on un-therapeutic behaviors, such as "questioning", thus producing an interview situation or "social conversation" consisting of actively taking part in the patient's life by bestowing praise, providing considerations, or taking a stand with regard to the patient's conflicts. The final group, with anti-therapeutic dynamics, referred to therapists embodying attitudes and behaviors with a negative or confusing function that had a harmful effect both on patient and therapist. For most novice therapists, concluded Killingmo et al. (2014), performing psychodynamic therapy seemed to demand a long learning rate.

To sum up, the results of these outcome studies indicate that therapists' personality is not easily changed. The adherence to a manual may lead to deterioration in interaction style, and difficulties in handling transference as well as countertransference may need a long period of supervised practice. The overall picture seems to be that novice trainees tend to be more in-and-out of an analytic attitude in sessions, whereas more experienced trainees tend to vary in degree of specific psychodynamic competencies. Concerning learning to work in the transference, we will claim that neither of these study designs were rigged for documenting the corresponding complex changes assumed to take place in a trainee when learning to work in the transference.

*Transferences in supervision – a challenge in the learning process*

Supervision plays a key role in the learning to work in the transference. What can results from empirical studies tell us about this learning process?

Feelings of incompetence and performance anxiety are typical for most trainee therapists (e.g., Orlinsky & Rønnestad, 2005; Rønnestad & Skovholt, 2013). This may hinder learning and create difficulties in understanding the patient's transference (e.g., Szecsödy, 1990). Moreover, the vulnerable position of the trainee paves the way for transference reactions toward the supervisor. As the supervisor is supposed to help, the feelings related to how the trainee has experienced to be helped by significant others prior in life is unavoidably activated. The overall and at the time unpredicted result in Doehrman's (1976) longitudinal interview study was that trainees develop intense relationships to their supervisors. Later, this result has been replicated without exceptions (e.g., Cabaniss et al., 2001; Carlsson, 2012; Nagell et al., 2014; Norberg et al., 2016; Strømme, 2012; Strømme, 2014; Strømme & Gullestad, 2012; Szecsödy, 1990; Wallerstein, 1981).

Does the quality of the supervision relationship change during training? In a longitudinal study based on audiotape-recorded supervision sessions and interviews, Szecsödy (1990) found that all the supervisees remained insecure and vulnerable during the whole training period. Both supervisees and supervisors tended to react defensively toward each other, concretized by being vague, too supportive, or too critical (pp. 143–144). None of the supervision couples developed more emotional openness and alliance.

In contrast to Szecsödy's results, Strømme (2012), in an interview study of pre-graduate psychologists, found that almost all the supervisees initially had strong negative feelings toward the supervisor, but that such feelings diminished during the one-year training. In a follow-up one year later, the picture was turned upside-down: Most of the supervisees expressed overall gratitude toward the supervisor. Surprisingly, the supervisors did not pick up the initial negative feelings, or at least not the extent of such feelings. In a sub-study, Strømme and Gullestad (2012) showed how one of the supervisees became less defensive and more openly exposed his own vulnerability during the process. Afterward, he questioned his own negative attitudes toward the supervisor initially and related them to lack of patience for the supervision relationship to unfold, as well as to transference reactions in himself. However, as for most of the other supervisees in the study, he never talked to the supervisor about these feelings. In another sub-study of two supervisees, transference reactions toward their supervisors were interpreted as activation of different kinds of negative object relations in these trainees (Strømme, 2014).

Supervisees' defensive reactions were also at the foreground in a survey study of psychoanalytic candidates (Cabaniss et al. 2001) revealing that half of the candidates reported anxiety about receiving credit for cases, which they typically did not talk about to the supervisor. In over half of the cases, neither the supervisor nor the supervisee addressed their relationship. Overall, the candidates reported high satisfaction, but 25% wanted to change supervisor, and 75% believed that such a switch would be labeled problematic. In contrast, over 75% of the supervisors reported that changing supervisors was unproblematic, indicating supervisee cautiousness.

How can supervisors handle strong negative feelings in supervisees? Doehrman (1976) concluded that becoming aware of the interpersonal processes in the therapeutic as well as in the supervision relationship instigated insights into the intrapsychic dynamics of both trainee and supervisor. Additionally, it enabled trainees, through model learning of the supervisor's handling in the situation, to address negative interactions in the therapy relationship, clearly fostering the trainees' abilities to work in the transference.

In a cross-sectional study, Zaslavsky et al. (2005) interviewed supervisors and psychoanalytic candidates. All supervisors exposed their own countertransference reactions toward the candidate to help them in discovering their contribution to qualities in the therapy relationship. The supervisors worked to find a suitable balance between what to address in supervision and what to leave for the personal analysis of the candidates.

Based on longitudinal interviews with four psychoanalytic candidates and their supervisors, Kantrowitz (2002) explored the characteristics of beneficial relationship matches. In three of the cases with character and style differences in the dyad, she found that the supervisors compensated for "an area of need in the candidate that was stimulated by the particular patient" (p. 964). Sometimes these compensations were first comprehended by the supervisees retrospectively and in these instances, not consciously realized by the supervisors. If the supervisees identified the compensation of the supervisor, they did not expose this understanding in the supervision. Moreover, Kantrowitz described how these supervisor compensations came to expression in the supervisee's therapeutic work in the form of an attitude, stance, or style. She stressed the idiosyncrasies of these processes.

Results of a single-case study (Leibovich & Zilcha-Mano, 2016) indicate that the supervisor's management of her own feelings toward the supervisee, and working through of own mistakes, can contribute to the quality of the supervisory relationship and the development of psychodynamic skills.

In a cross-sectional survey with psychoanalytic candidates and supervisors, Nagell et al. (2014) found that both parts agreed that their relationship was not much explored during the supervisory work. In two of four groups describing the supervisees reactions to the supervisors interventions, the supervisees reacted in a phobic-avoidant or a reserved-adaptive style, avoiding a focus on their relational capacities. This is in opposition to supervisees wanting this focus, which was the largest supervisee group, and supervisors with supervisees wanting such a focus, both of these groups rated highest on the supervisees' development of a psychoanalytic identity. These supervisees were also more satisfied with the supervision. We may ask if the results indicate that positive transferences were activated in these candidates toward the supervisor and vice versa for candidates not wanting a focus on the relationship. However, there is a positive trend during the supervision process; dyads at advanced training level were more satisfied with the supervision and evaluated the therapy and the training outcome more highly compared to beginners, in line with the positive developmental process found by Strømme and Gullestad (2012).

"Parallel processes" refer to instances where dynamics in the therapy relationship can appear in the supervision relationship, or vice versa, as a kind of unconscious communication between the participants (e.g., Doehrman, 1976; Fleming & Benedek, 1966). Several studies (e.g., Caligor, 1981; Friedlander et al., 1989; Raichelson et al., 1997) have addressed parallel-process phenomena, but today, the perspective has lost much of its significance. Critics have stated that what may overtly seem like the same intrapsychic dynamics more likely relates to divergent intrapsychic processes in the participants (c.p., Watkins, 2017).

In sum, trainees typically have transference- and defensive reactions toward their supervisor. Such reactions are difficult to handle while a complex and challenging learning process is going on. Most studies support addressing such reactions in supervision. However, trainees may also feel mastery by being able to understand and handle intense emotions by themselves. Others may not trust the supervisor enough to explore their own vulnerabilities. Only a couple of studies document changes in supervisees' defensive reactions and relational patterns. In our view, an important limitation is that the referred studies are based primarily on data from the supervision process and don't include data from the therapy process. In total, the studies, shifting between a bird-view perspective and detailed idiosyncratic descriptions, give a rather fragmented description of the inner learning process and the outcome of the trainees.

## Discussion

What can be concluded about empirical research on trainee change? First, there are no studies specifically analyzing learning to work in the transference, and surprisingly little empirical research during the last decades has addressed the issue one way or another. Moreover, in line with the general picture in training research (Hill & Knox, 2013; Knox & Hill, 2021; Watkins, 2020), the studies are also limited in numbers and characterized by conceptual and methodological limitations. Furthermore, within the psychodynamic tradition, there is no consensus about how to define pivotal concepts such as transference and countertransference (Tuckett, 2005). One possibility is to rely on either participants' or expert evaluators' own understanding of the relevant concepts (e.g., the "Consensual Qualitative Research (CQR) model" (Hill et al., 2005)); both approaches are highly relevant when trying to analyze transference and countertransference phenomena based on interview data and recorded sessions.

Moreover, we do not know for sure to what extent therapist skills can be learned at all. Recent studies convincingly show that some therapists achieve better outcomes than others (Castonguay & Hill, 2017; Wampold & Owen, 2021). However, research indicates that more effective therapists are characterized by sophisticated interpersonal skills that are likely rooted in their personal lives and attachment history (Heinonen & Nissen-Lie, 2020).

There may also be limitations in the way we train. Bion's seminal book *Learning from Experience* (1962) has ever since been referred to as a key to psychodynamic understanding of learning. Bion (1962) states that we need another person's mind to help us endure the anxiety that is awakened in us. When our affects are contained by another, they gradually can be tolerated, enabling psychological processing and symbolization. However, the new deliberate-practice tradition in general psychotherapy training argues that we must implement components from expertise training in other professions, such as sports, pilot training, music, and medicine (Ericsson, 2018). Preliminary studies indicate that procedural training can lead to better patient outcomes (Chow et al., 2015; Goldberg et al., 2016) and increased clinical skills (Anderson et al., 2020; Hill et al., 2020; Perlman et al., 2020; Westra et al., 2021). Can such a training approach be combined with Bion's idea of containment to perform the complex task of working in the transference? Or will it be yet another kind of a manual-based training approach with the same limitations as found in the Vanderbilt II study? These questions remain to be investigated.

### A new study of learning to work in the transference

Because of the shortages in the transference-training research, we have developed a study of learning to work in the transference. This longitudinal sub-study is part of the larger research project NORTRAS.

Our research question is:

During the corresponding therapy and supervision processes, how does a psychology student at the internal practicum in the last year of a six-year professional-oriented study program in psychology learn to contain and intervene in the transference here-and-now in the therapy relationship with the help of supervision?

We have collected video data from both psychotherapy and supervision. We have started a single-case study looking into all videos of the psychotherapy and supervision sessions of one therapist. The results of this study will be used as a blueprint for qualitative analysis across different cases.

We will attain relevant data to compare how transference is addressed and worked with in therapy as well as in supervision. In the analysis of the video recordings, we are using reflective thematic analysis (Braun &

Clarke, 2019). We complement this analysis with filled-in questionnaires and a combination of semi-structured and interpersonal-process recall interviews (Kagan, 1984) with the trainee, the supervisor, and the patient. The focus is permanently on the trainee, but the contributions of the supervisor and the patient are also included. As a validation step, OPD analyses are performed. The Operationalised Psychodynamic Diagnostic System (OPD-3, 2023) with its four axes enables exposing of structural levels of the personality, as well as inner unconscious conflicts.

As transference work is a specific skill, data analysis is not a bottom-up process in a strict sense. Instead, it is informed by our own psychoanalytic understanding of transference-countertransference phenomena, object-relational theory, affect theories, and by the OPD results.

We do not claim to determine what is going on within the therapists during training. Instead, we may add additional options and suggestions for interpretations, which link observable behavior with inner phenomena in order to investigate the development of this skill in a more detailed way.

## Conclusion

There is only fragmented empirical research on the change process taking place in trainees during learning to work in the transference. Further empirical research is not only needed to investigate the learning process in more detail and for developing the psychoanalytic therapeutic tradition further. Better studies are also required in order to test main assumptions and to substantiate the relevance of significant concepts and the effects of crucial therapeutic skills, such as working with transference-countertransference.

## Note

1  We include both studies of psychoanalytic and psychodynamic training but for simplicity, we will from now on use psychoanalytic competence when referring to being able to work in the transference.

## References

Anderson, T., Perlman, M. R., McCarrick, S. M., & McClintock, A. S. (2020). Modeling therapist responses with structured practice enhances facilitative interpersonal skills. *Journal of Clinical Psychology*, 76(4), 659–675.

Arbeitskreis OPD (Hrsg.). (2023). *OPD-3 - Operationalisierte psychodynamische diagnostik*. Hogrefe.

Bion, W. R. (1962). *Learning from experience*. Karnac Books Ltd.

Braun, V., & V. Clarke (2019). Reflecting on reflexive thematic analysis. *Qualitative Research in Sport, Exercise and Health*, 11(4), 589–597.

Buckley, P., Conte, H. R., Plutchik, R, Karasu, T. B. & Wild, K. V. (1982). Learning dynamic psychotherapy: A longitudinal study. *The American Journal of Psychiatry*, 139, 1607–1610.

Cabaniss, D. L., Glick, R. A., & Roose, S. P. (2001). The Columbia supervision project: Data from the dyad. *Journal of the American Psychoanalytic Association, 49*(1), 235–267.

Caligor, L. (1981). Parallel and reciprocal processes in psychoanalytic supervision. *Contemporary Psychoanalysis, 17*, 1–27.

Carlsson, J. (2012). Research on psychotherapists' professional development during and after training. *Nordic Psychology, 64*, 150–167.

Castonguay, L. G., & Hill, C. E. (Eds.). (2017). *How and why are some therapists better than others? Understanding therapist effects.* American Psychological Association.

Chow, D. L., Miller, S. D., Seidel, J. A., Kane, R. T., Thornton, J. A., & Andrews, W. P. (2015). The role of deliberate practice in the development of highly effective psychotherapists. *Psychotherapy, 52*(3), 337–345.

Doehrman, M. J. (1976). Parallel processes in supervision and psychotherapy. *Bulletin of the Menninger Clinic, 40*(1), 3–104.

Ericsson, K. A. (2018). The differential influence of experience, practice, and deliberate practice on the development of superior individual performance of experts. In K. A. Ericsson, R. R. Hoffman, A. Kozbelt, & A. M. Williams (Eds.), *The Cambridge handbook of expertise and expert performance* (pp. 745–769). Cambridge University Press.

Fleming, J., & Benedek, T. F. (1966). *Psychoanalytic supervision. A method of clinical teaching.* Grune & Stratton.

Friedlander, M. L., Siegel, S. M., & Brenock, K. (1989). Parallel process in counseling and supervision: A case study. *Journal of Counseling Psychology, 36*(2), 149–157.

Goldberg, S. B., Rousmaniere, T., Miller, S. D., Whipple, J., Nielsen, S. L., Hoyt, W. T., & Wampold, B. E. (2016). Do psychotherapists improve with time and experience? A longitudinal analysis of outcomes in a clinical setting. *Journal of Counseling Psychology, 63*(1), 1–11.

Gullestad, S. E., & B. Killingmo (2020). *The theory and practice of psychoanalytic therapy. Listening for the subtext.* Routledge.

Heinonen, E., & Nissen-Lie, H. A. (2020). The professional and personal characteristics of effective psychotherapists: A systematic review. *Psychotherapy Research, 30*(4), 417–432.

Henry, W P., Strupp, H. H., Butler, S. E, Schacht, T. E., & Binder, J. L. (1993). Effects of training in time-limited dynamic psychotherapy: Changes in therapist behavior. *Journal of Consulting and Clinical Psychology, 61*, 434–440.

Hill, C. E., Baumann, E., Shafran, N., Gupta, S., Morrison, A., Rojas, A. E. P., ... & Gelso, C. J. (2015). Is training effective? A study of counseling psychology doctoral trainees in a psychodynamic/interpersonal training clinic. *Journal of Counseling Psychology, 62*(2), 184–201.

Hill, C. E., Kivlighan III, D. M., Rousmaniere, T., Kivlighan, D. M., Jr., Gerstenblith, J. A., & Hillman, J. W. (2020). Deliberate practice for the skill of immediacy: A multiple case study of doctoral student therapists and clients. *Psychotherapy, 57*(4), 587–597.

Hill, C. E., & Knox, S. (2013). Training and supervision in psychotherapy. In M. J. Lambert (Ed.), *Bergin and Garfield's handbook of psychotherapy and behavior change* (pp. 775–811). John Wiley & Sons.

Hill, C. E., Knox, S., Thompson, B. J., Williams, E. N., Hess, S. A., & Ladany, N. (2005). Consensual qualitative research: An update. *Journal of counseling psychology, 52*(2), 196–205.

Hilsenroth, M. J., Defife, J. A., Blagys, M. D., & Ackerman, S. J. (2006). Effects of training in short-term psychodynamic psychotherapy: Changes in graduate clinician technique. *Psychotherapy Research*, *16*(03), 293–305.

Kagan, N. (1984). Interpersonal process recall: Basic methods and recent research. In D. Larson (Ed.), *Teaching psychological skills: Models for giving psychology away* (pp. 229–244). Brooks/Cole.

Kantrowitz, J. L. (2002). The triadic match: The interactive effect of supervisor, candidate, and patient. *Journal of the American Psychoanalytic Association*, *50*(3), 939–968.

Killingmo, B., Varvin, S., & Strømme, H. (2014). What can we expect from trainee therapists? A study of acquisition of competence in dynamic psychotherapy. *Scandinavian Psychoanalytic Review*, *37*(1), 24–35.

Knox, S., & Hill, C. E. (2021). Training and supervision in psychotherapy: What we know and where we need to go. In M. Barkham, W. Lutz, & L. G. Castonguay (Eds.), *Begin and Garfield's handbook of psychotherapy and behavior change* (pp. 327–349). Wiley.

Leibovich, L., & Zilcha-Mano, S. (2016). What is the right time for supportive versus expressive interventions in supervision? An illustration based on a clinical mistake. *Psychotherapy*, *53*(3), 297–301.

Nagell, W., Steinmetzer, L., Fissabre, U., & Spilski, J. (2014). Research into the relationship experience in supervision and its influence on the psychoanalytical identity formation of candidate trainees. *Psychoanalytic Inquiry*, *34*(6), 554–583.

Norberg, J., Axelsson, H., Barkman, N., Hamrin, M., & Carlsson, J. (2016). What psychodynamic supervisors say about supervision: Freedom within limits. *The Clinical Supervisor*, *35*(2), 268–286.

Orlinsky, D. E., & Rønnestad, M. H. (2005). *How psychotherapists develop: A study of therapeutic work and professional growth*. American Psychological Association.

Perlman, M. R., Anderson, T., Foley, V. K., Mimnaugh, S., & Safran, J. D. (2020). The impact of alliance-focused and facilitative interpersonal relationship training on therapist skills: An RCT of brief training. *Psychotherapy Research*, *30*(7), 871–884.

Raichelson, S. H., Herron, W. G., Primavera, L. H., & Ramirez, S. M. (1997). Incidence and effects of parallel process in psychotherapy supervision. *The Clinical Supervisor*, *15*(2), 37–48.

Ravitz, P., Lawson, A., Fefergrad, M., Rawkins, S., Lancee, W., Maunder, R., ... & Kivlighan, D. M. (2019). Psychotherapy competency milestones: An exploratory pilot of CBT and psychodynamic psychotherapy skills acquisition in junior psychiatry residents. *Academic Psychiatry*, *43*, 61–66.

Rønnestad, M. H., & Skovholt, T. M. (2013). *The developing practitioner: Growth and stagnation of therapists and counselors*. Routledge.

Strømme, H. (2012). Confronting helplessness: A study of the acquisition of dynamic psychotherapeutic competence by psychology students. *Nordic Psychology*, *64*(3), 203–217.

Strømme, H. (2014). A bad and a better supervision process; actualized relational scenarios in trainees: A longitudinal study of nondisclosure in psychodynamic supervision. *Psychoanalytic Inquiry*, *34*(6), 584–605.

Strømme, H., & Gullestad, S. E. (2012). Disclosure or non-disclosure? An in-depth study of psychodynamic supervision. *The Scandinavian Psychoanalytic Review*, *35*(2), 105–115.

Szecsödy, I. (1990). *The learning process in psychotherapy supervision*. Department of Psychiatry, Karolinska Institutet, St Görans Hospital.

Tuckett, D. (2005). Does anything go? Towards a framework for the more transparent assessment of psychoanalytic competence. *International Journal of Psychoanalytic, 86*, 31–49.

Wallerstein, R. S. (Ed.). (1981). *Becoming a psychoanalyst. A study of psychoanalytic supervision*. International Universities Press.

Wampold, B. E., & Owen, J. (2021). Therapist effects: History, methods, magnitude, and characteristics of effective therapists. In M. Barkham, W. Lutz, & L. G. Castonguay (Eds.), *Begin and Garfield's handbook of psychotherapy and behavior change* (pp. 297–326). Wiley.

Watkins Jr, C. E. (2017). Reconsidering parallel process in psychotherapy supervision: On parsimony, rival hypotheses, and alternate explanations. *Psychoanalytic Psychology, 34*(4), 506–515.

Watkins Jr, C. E. (2020). What do clinical supervision research reviews tell us? Surveying the last 25 years. *Counseling Psychotherapy Research, 20*, 190–208.

Westra, H. A., Norouzian, N., Poulin, L., Coyne, A., Constantino, M. J., Hara, K., … & Antony, M. M. (2021). Testing a deliberate practice workshop for developing appropriate responsivity to resistance markers. *Psychotherapy, 58*(2), 175–185.

Zaslavsky, J., Nunes, M. L. T., & Eizirik, C. L. (2005). Approaching countertransference in psychoanalytical supervision: A qualitative investigation. *The International Journal of Psychoanalysis, 86*(4), 1099–1131.

# 17 A microanalytic method to investigate psychoanalytic process

## In search of the in-between

*Carolina Altimir and Juan Pablo Jiménez*

### Introduction

This chapter argues in favor of establishing a constructive dialogue between science and hermeneutics in psychoanalysis to address the question of what defines psychoanalytic process, a question subject of a constant and ongoing debate. After 100 years, the psychoanalytic movement still does not reach an agreement about what true psychoanalysis is (Jiménez & Altimir, 2019). Although theory and practice of psychoanalysis have been influenced by postmodernism and its notion of the existence of different conceptions of psychoanalysis, and rejection of authoritarian positions, there remains a strong dichotomy between those who adopt an eminently hermeneutic stance in the generation of knowledge about psychoanalytic process, and those who incorporate the contributions of science and systematic observation. Thus, theoretical and empirical pluralism is a pathway toward addressing this dichotomy; insofar practical and theoretical diversity are inevitable in psychoanalysis when attempting to explain complex phenomena. This implies opening psychoanalysis to an active and mutually enriching dialogue with related disciplines as well as with empirical research (Jiménez & Altimir, 2019).

### The centrality of the concept "psychoanalytic process"

When attempting to define what is essentially psychoanalytic in a particular psychotherapeutic treatment, there is consensus in pointing to the analytic process as the most prominent feature. However, after important efforts within the psychoanalytic community to develop a consensual definition, no agreement has been achieved regarding what transpires between patient and analyst within the analytic session that can be defined as psychoanalytic process (Tuckett, 2004). The final conclusion is that each analytic process is unique, ideographic, and therefore different and incomparable to any other, or to any other analytic dyad (Foehl, 2010).

DOI: 10.4324/9781032651934-22

*Traditional psychoanalytic inquiry*

The traditional source of psychoanalytic knowledge has been clinical inquiry, characterized by the adoption of a hermeneutic stance, where understanding is attained through interpretation of the other's experience and reality. Understanding through interpretation implies embracing complexity, that is, being aware that our comprehension of a phenomena will always be incomplete, given the natural limitations of our understanding (Orange, 2011). From the point of view of the hermeneutic task, the understanding of the unique individual is also the understanding of its context (Gadamer, 1966). As Irvin Hoffman (2009) asserts, the analyst accepts the existential uncertainty that accompanies the realization that there are multiple good ways to be and that the individual's choices are always influenced by culture, personal values, countertransference, and other factors in ways that can never be fully known. For many analysts who embrace this perspective, any attempt that seeks to answer the question of analytic process based on empirical research is considered reductionist and therefore threatens to ignore its essentially indeterminate and unique character (McWilliams, 2011; Wallerstein, 1993).

At the same time, the primary means by which traditional psychoanalytic inquiry communicates and reports its insights and formulations on analytic process is case studies (Kächele et al., 2009; Kächele et al., 2012). Although clinical vignettes have contributed enormously in the development of theory since Freud, being the source of important clinical hypotheses, they have often lacked a systematic procedure that accounts for how the information is selected and communicated. Vignettes are often selected by the therapist – who is involved in the process – based on his/her theoretical predilections and with the purpose of emphasizing and supporting a specific formulation (Grünbaum, 1984). It is important to note that the analyst's subjective position in relation to the object of study is not a problem in itself, as extensive qualitative research has taught us (McLeod, 2011). What is problematic is to not state this position and its underlying assumptions as part of the investigator's contribution to the inquiry process, a measure that safeguards methodological integrity (Levitt, 2020). Thus, the criteria and procedures for the selection of the material are not available for scrutiny by the clinical and scientific community (Messer, 2007) and therefore cannot be susceptible of being interrogated by different actors, and reaching alternative plausible explanations of the phenomenon (Fonagy & Moran, 1993).

*The relational turn in psychoanalysis*

Contemporary understanding of the psychoanalytic process has been influenced by the relational turn, which has reached nearly all psychoanalytic schools of thought (Bohleber, 2013). This movement has reconceptualized traditional psychoanalytic theory and practice based on the premise that relationships with others are the basic matter of mental life. Its basic unit of study is not the individual as a separate entity whose desires collide with an external reality, but an interactional field within which the individual emerges and struggles to come into contact and articulate – thus, the mind is composed of relational configurations (Mitchell, 1988). Psychoanalytic process is therefore understood as all that transpires within this relational matrix between analyst and patient, where their subjective experiences influence one another (Aron, 1996), requiring a mutual negotiation that needs to deal with both participants' needs for self-agency and relatedness (Safran & Muran, 2000).

Noteworthy, the relational turn has been greatly influenced by mother–infant research and affect regulation theory – extra-clinical findings based on systematic research. The advances in the field of developmental psychology, neuroscience, and attachment have gathered substantial evidence indicating the interactive nature of the development of the human mind and brain (Schore, 2003). These findings suggest that the self develops within a relational matrix through processes that are organized dyadically between the infant and its caregiver (Schore, 2016). Affect is transacted within the infant–caregiver exchange through a highly efficient and essentially non-verbal system of emotional communication (Allen, 2013). Affect regulation constitutes, then, a central mechanism in the process through which the infant moves from a primary state of co-regulation with its caregiver toward self-regulation, laying the foundations of the development of the self (Fonagy et al., 2002); thus, it is a central organizing principle of human development and motivation (Schore, 2003).

Hence, the centrality of affect as the currency of the relational configurations that form the basis for the development of the self has been incorporated into the relational conceptualization of human development and psychoanalytic process in contemporary relational psychoanalytic thought. The emotional exchange between patient and therapist becomes an essential element of the therapeutic endeavor, and affect regulation in particular can be thought of as a mechanism involved in psychotherapeutic change, insofar as adaptive exchanges create an opportunity to reorganize and acquire new repertoires of affective negotiation (Safran & Muran, 2000).

Here, we can witness an advancement in the attempt to better define psychoanalytic process. Nevertheless, this conceptualization is based on the transfer of the basic principles – derived from empirical research – that guide mother–infant transactions, to the adult analytic situation. Although they have contributed to an enormous development of clinical hypotheses and understanding, the field is still in debt in terms of generating knowledge about psychoanalysis by studying the psychoanalytic process itself.

*Outcome and process-outcome research in psychotherapy and psychoanalysis*

Around the same time, a group of eminent psychoanalytic researchers adopted systematic research as a method to acquire knowledge on psychoanalysis and validate it within the scientific community. One line of research focused on undergoing outcomes studies to prove that psychoanalysis and psychoanalytic therapy were effective (De Maat et al., 2013; Leichsenring, 2005). While important in justifying the value of psychoanalytic treatment to society, however, these types of studies say nothing about the processes and mechanisms of therapeutic change and do not illuminate psychoanalytic practice.

In an effort to examine the relationship between psychoanalytic process and the final results of therapy, another group of psychoanalytic researchers adopted the process-outcome approach to psychotherapy research, which has proven relevant in advancing knowledge on how psychotherapy works. This approach examines change processes – what takes place during therapy sessions – as well as mechanisms occurring within the patient that are associated with treatment outcome (Crits-Christoph & Connolly Gibbons, 2021). Researchers, such as Luborsky, Spence, Vaughan, Dahl, and Ablon and Jones, viewed the need to incorporate empirical research methods to the study of psychoanalytic process, in order to generate systematic knowledge, offering ideas, concepts, and measurement approaches. Thomä, Kächele, and Ulm's group investigated the psychoanalytic process systematically with empirical methodology for forty years. Although they have contributed to a more precise knowledge about psychoanalytic treatment, Tuckett, in 2004, asserted that psychoanalytic process still eludes definition and now, despite a good deal of psychoanalytic research, we cannot identify substantial progress in empirically validating the concept of psychoanalytic process. Schachter and Kächele (2017) conclude that we have reached a stalemate, where it is not possible either to define or to measure the traditional concept of "psychoanalytic process" and propose therefore to change strategies and focus on a detailed observation and description of the analyst–patient interaction using modern technologies such as videotaping.

## Proposing a clinically sensitive empirical research paradigm in psychoanalysis

A clinically sensitive empirical research approach to studying psychoanalytic process that builds on the previously discussed issues is proposed. It adopts epistemological and methodological pluralism to develop a dialogue between hermeneutics and science, under the guiding question of *which method of research – clinical, empirical, quantitative or qualitative, conceptual, etc. – can be used to brighten which particular psychoanalytic problem or question?* (Altimir & Jiménez, 2020). This implies building on findings from varying related disciplines and assumes the premises that guide general psychotherapy process-outcome research, that is, the need to enrich an "evidence-based therapeutic practice" beyond "brands", and contribute to answer the question of "what works for whom" under what circumstances, based on the observation and examination of what really takes place within therapeutic process and how this is linked to therapy outcome. We can learn more about the psychoanalytic process by studying the process itself. It is the path to link theory-driven "top-down" research, guided by psychoanalytic concepts, and "bottom-up" research that does justice to real psychoanalytic practice.

This research approach is a pathway for the examination of psychoanalytic process. It is clinically sensitive, as it is interested in examining two main elements that are considered relevant for analytic process: the dyadic and interpersonal relevance of the patient–analyst encounter and the implicit (unformulated) domain of this exchange in relation to the symbolic dimension of experience. To address the first dimension, the basic study unit is defined as the analytic relationship, with a focus on "the in-between." This definition relies on relational concepts of human development and of the psychotherapeutic situation as organizing conceptual models of the phenomenon under study. The guiding principles for addressing the dimension of implicit, unconscious experience within this interactive unit are the contributions from affective neurosciences, neuropsychoanalysis, mother–infant research, and research on non-verbal human behavior. Given the methodological challenge of studying these phenomena, the strategy is to resort to the observation of behavior that can give access to such unconscious processes (i.e., facial affective behavior) (Altimir & Jiménez, 2020).

A flexible combination of three methodological approaches is proposed to achieve this. First, the implementation of cumulative systematic case studies (Messer, 2007), since the interest is both in accounting for the uniqueness of each analytic process, and deriving common principles based on systematic observation of repeated and characteristic patterns of experience. Second, the adoption of the events paradigm as an approach to the study of the therapy process (Safran, 2003). It is based on systematic observation of salient events within therapy sessions that constitute "thick" experiential instances which concentrate meaningful information about the mechanisms that are most significant for the analytical process (Safran, 2003). Third, a micro-analytic approach to the specific phenomena occurring within relevant sequences of the patient–analyst interaction, which provide access to implicit and unconscious dimensions that are otherwise overlooked by approaches based on broader units of analysis. These three methodological approaches can be combined as different but complementary lenses into the analytic process, where patterns, behaviors, and mechanisms that are described at one level of analysis are contextualized and signified by the processes and mechanisms that simultaneously take place at the other levels of observation (Altimir & Jiménez, 2020).

### Ongoing research process: building bridges between the unformulated-unconscious and the explicit-formulated edges in psychoanalytic process research

The research program described above has been implemented by a research group in the study of affect regulation between patient and therapist as a clinically relevant component of psychotherapeutic process in general and of analytic process in particular (Altimir & Jiménez, 2021). The concept of affect regulation stands at the crossroads of cognitive neuroscience, developmental psychology, attachment, etiopathogenesis, personality, psychopathology, psychiatry, and psychotherapy, given its relevance for both adaptive and maladaptive mental functioning (Altimir et al., 2021). This is a concept stemming from related disciplines that is of great value for psychoanalytic process, insofar as relational psychoanalytic literature highlights the notion of intersubjective negotiation of affective states and needs between patient and therapist (Aron, 1996).

The study of affect regulation initiated within a single case of psychodynamic brief psychotherapy (Altimir & Valdés-Sánchez, 2020). Progressively, the study of five new brief psychotherapies was included (mostly psychoanalytic-oriented). Currently, a total of 15 psychotherapeutic processes have been included in a progressively growing sample of cases. All studies have adopted the events paradigm to examine affect regulation within the therapeutic process. In accordance with the conceptual framework guiding the program's understanding of relational phenomena, the studies draw on Safran and Muran's (2000; Muran et al., 2022) *Rupture Resolution Model* to select the specific in-session events that would "concentrate" relevant features of patient–therapist affect regulation. Safran and Muran (2000) proposed a dynamic notion of the therapeutic alliance in which a continuous negotiation – both interpersonal and intrapsychic, conscious and unconscious – takes place within the therapist–patient dyad. The interpersonal level involves a negotiation between the subjectivities of patient and therapist; the intrapsychic level involves the negotiation between the patient's needs for agency and relatedness. The tensions, conscious or unconscious, experienced on these dimensions manifest themselves through ruptures. Ruptures can induce emotional distress and activate relational and self-schemas commanded by the characteristic patterns of coping with stress, thus eliciting the domain of affect regulation (self- and hetero-regulation) (Muran et al., 2022).

Ruptures can manifest as confrontations and as withdrawals. Confrontations are more direct and involve a manifestation of disagreement or concern with the therapy or therapist. Withdrawals involve the patient distancing from the therapist or the therapeutic process, by denying an aspect of him/herself to appease the therapist. Withdrawal ruptures tend to prioritize the need for relatedness over agency, while confrontation ruptures tend to indicate a patient's difficulties expressing relational needs, therefore favoring agency (Muran & Eubanks, 2020). Meanwhile, timely and appropriate repair of ruptures are associated with therapeutic change, as they allow the patient to explore, challenge, and change maladaptive interpersonal patterns and develop more flexible and adaptive ways of negotiating needs in a relationship (Safran & Muran, 2000).

Within the therapeutic exchange, patient and analyst experience and regulate internal affective states, expressing them through verbal and non-verbal channels. For accessing the implicit-unconscious domain of experience, the study resorts to micro-analytic examination of patient and therapist facial-affective behavior. Findings from research on facial expression of emotions (Ekman, 2007) and facial-affective behavior in psychotherapy (Benecke & Krause, 2005) indicate that facial affective behavior is an observable component of emotional processes that is organized at a non-symbolic, non-verbal, unconscious level and to which both members of the dyad react beneath awareness. Affective processes are inherent to the therapeutic exchange, and relevant instances of this exchange trigger varying degrees of emotional dysregulation in the dyad, with their concomitant attempts to self- and mutual regulation. In this context, each emotion implies a specific desire for regulation and, when expressed, constitutes a specific relational offer to the interactive partner (Benecke & Krause, 2005). These communications are carried out at an implicit level of signaling and response that occur too rapidly for simultaneous verbal translation and conscious reflection (Lyons-Ruth, 2000); however, they are captured and used to evaluate, assess, and regulate relationships, communicate internal emotional states, and regulate affect.

Patient and therapists' facial affective behavior within ruptures and resolution attempts was examined. These events provide a context of meaning that can make sense of the "smaller" descriptions derived from facial micro-analysis. They adopt a communicative value within that specific relational context, serving as information about the interactive partner's experience and therefore influencing the concomitant affective response (Altimir & Jiménez, 2021).

These studies proceeded to videotape all therapy sessions using two separate video cameras installed in each treatment room, each recording the upper torso and face/head of each member of the therapeutic dyad. Subsequently, expert judges observed each session video, assisted with the session verbatim transcript and identified rupture and resolution strategy, based on the Rupture Resolution System (Eubanks et al., 2015). After that, video segments of rupture and resolution strategies were analyzed by trained coders using the Facial Action Coding System (Ekman & Friesen, 1978). This system allows the objective coding of two types of facial-affective behaviors, which, based on previous research, have been considered to have specific regulatory functions (self- and hetero-regulation). The first group are basic emotions (happiness, anger, contempt, disgust, fear, sadness, and surprise), which not only communicate to the person's intra-psychic emotional state but, at the same time, conveys a certain meaning that is directed toward the interactive partner: a desire for hetero-regulation of the emotional state, an evaluation of the object of reference. The second group are non-specific facial actions, indicators of emotional arousal, and attempts at regulation: (1) gaze behavior (directing gaze toward the interactive partner, or averting gaze), which regulates emotional involvement in the interaction and the direction of the expressed affect; (2) face self-touching (indicators of emotional tension or arousal and the attempt at self-regulation); (3) control/attenuation of expressions (movements around the mouth that indicate self-regulation of the expression); and (4) elevation of the eyebrows (conveys emphasis or interrogation) (Altimir & Valdés-Sánchez, 2020).

The study units are nested within each other: patient and therapist's facial behavior takes place within the same dyad that is negotiating their relationship, expressed in ruptures and resolution strategy episodes. In turn, these episodes take place within the therapy sessions. Finally, therapy sessions take place within the therapy as a whole and may have different characteristics depending on their location within this process: beginning, middle, and end of therapy. Therefore, the likelihood that patient and therapist display certain facial affective behaviors is inevitably influenced by their particular relationship and the ruptures and resolution strategies they co-create, which are in turn influenced by the phase of the therapy process. Therefore, statistical nested data analyses have been carried out.

### Initial results: what can we say so far?

Based on the overall results of this program, it is possible to establish that there are characteristic patient–therapist facial-verbal regulatory patterns for both ruptures and resolution strategies.

An initial set of results are based on a single case study of a brief psychoanalytic psychotherapy. Findings indicate that during ruptures, the patient conveyed signs of emotional dysregulation and displayed negative emotions (fear and anger), as well as control processes of the emotions, indicating emotional disturbance. She also gazed away from the therapist, although she expressed a receptive attitude in her verbalizations. The therapist showed a tendency to maintain contact and involvement with the patient through gaze behavior directed toward her, despite manifesting markers of emotional dysregulation and control.

Meanwhile, during resolution strategies – when the therapist acknowledged the ruptures and made attempts at repairing them – the patient resumed contact with him through engaged gaze, showing involvement in the interaction, despite displaying indicators of emotional dysregulation. The therapist seemed to regulate himself while attempting repair, displaying facial behaviors indicative of him being empathetic and interrogative (Altimir & Valdés-Sánchez, 2020).

A second set of results derives from the analysis of five psychothera-pies in which only ruptures were analyzed, and the comparison was made between patient and therapist behavior. Therapists displayed significantly more signs of emotional dysregulation than their patients during ruptures, while maintaining their involvement in the interaction by continuously directing their gaze toward their patient. This behavior became more fre-quent when the patient gazed away. Meanwhile, patients manifested a marked tendency to avoid eye contact and therefore emotional and atten-tional involvement in the interaction with their therapist. This study goes further by examining participants' facial-affective behavior in withdrawal and confrontation ruptures. During withdrawal ruptures, patients show greater probability of expressing positive emotions through smiles, and establishing more eye contact than during confrontation ruptures. In this case, most withdrawal ruptures were of the type called content-affect dis-sociation, where patients withdraw from the therapist or the therapy work by exhibiting affects (often positive) that do not coincide with the content of their narrative (Barros et al, 2016).

A final set of results derive from the analysis of ruptures and resolution strategies belonging to thirteen brief psychotherapies and 227 therapy ses-sions. This yielded 242 ruptures and 76 resolution strategies. Preliminary analyses of a sample of these events have indicated that during ruptures, patients express significantly more positive (smile) and negative (fear, sad-ness, and disgust) emotions than during resolution strategies. At the same time, they display more facial-affective markers of emotional dysregulation and tend to conceal their affective expressions. However, contrary to the previous studies, the patients of this sample displayed more eye contact with their therapist during ruptures, compared with resolution strategies. This difference is explained by the fact that little or no resolution strategies were analyzed in the previous studies and that the type of statistical analy-sis is of a different nature.

Previous results are supported by this new study, which shows that pa-tients displayed more positive emotions during withdrawal ruptures (in which they are not explicit with their discomfort) and more negative emo-tions (mostly fear) in confrontation ruptures. This supports the notion that patients tend to privilege relational needs over agency during withdrawal ruptures, by "protecting" their bond with their therapist, through the ex-pression of positive emotions. Therapists also express more positive and negative emotions (fear and sadness), as well as more emotional dysregu-lation, during ruptures compared to resolution strategies. They show no differences in their facial behavior between withdrawal and confrontation ruptures and maintain eye contact and engagement with their patient at all times, confirming the results of the previous studies.

This last study has also examined the association of the presence of rup-tures and resolution strategies with therapeutic change, showing that ther-apies whose patients showed clinically significant improvement presented more withdrawal ruptures. Meanwhile, therapies whose patients did not achieve a clinically significant change, but maintained a functional level, presented more confrontation ruptures. These results are in line with previous findings in the field, suggesting that confrontation ruptures are related to lower therapeutic benefits. However, these findings need yet to be confirmed by further nested analyses of the entire sample of events.

### Closing remarks

This chapter has outlined a clinically sensitive research program proposal based on a bottom-up approach to describing and making sense of the psychoanalytic process. This type of research is a contribution to theory development as it allows the possibility of making new statements about analytic process, sustained on systematic observation on how psychotherapy is being carried out in routine practice. The systematic description of interactions belonging to the micro-level of the therapeutic endeavor constitutes an observable proxy of the elements and processes that are linked to psychoanalytic concepts of a higher order, but that can be connected to the moment-to-moment experience of the analytic interaction. In other words, clinicians may have in mind these observable sequences of interaction as indicators of higher ordered concepts and identify them in their practice as they take place, allowing an immediate and adequate intervention. Specifically, the domain of affect regulation serves the function of connecting interactions near to experience to higher ordered concepts that are relevant to psychoanalytic process.

Since this is still ongoing research, there are numerous questions that remain open, as well as severalideas of how these results may have implications for clinical practice, but due to space limitations, we have restricted ourselves to the research aspects of our model. Nevertheless, findings so far should be complemented with in-depth qualitative research exploring therapist's (and patients' if possible) subjective experience of these events, using methods of reconstructive observation of therapy segments. It is also important to extend our studies to long-term therapies since the characteristics of the overall therapy process are different. Finally, we must consider the limitations of the present research proposal in cases where the psychoanalytic setting is defined by the use of the couch, where there are no face-to-face interactions.

### References

Allen, J. G. (2013). *Restoring Mentalizing in Attachment Relationships. Treating Trauma with Plain Old Therapy*. Washington, DC: American Psychiatric Publishing.

Altimir, C., de la Cerda, C., & Dagnino, P. (2021). The functional domain of affect regulation. In G. de la Parra, P. Dagnino, & A. Behn (Eds.), *Depression and Personality Dysfunction. An Integrative Functional Domains Perspective* (pp. 33–70). Springer. doi:10.1007/978-3-030-70699-9.

Altimir, C., & Jiménez, J. P. (2020). Walking the middle ground between hermeneutics and science: A research proposal on psychoanalytic process. *The International Journal of Psychoanalysis, 101*(3), 496–522. doi:10.1080/00207578.2020.1726711.

Altimir, C., & Jiménez, J. P. (2021). The clinical relevance of interdisciplinary research on affect regulation in the analytic relationship. *Frontiers in Psychology.* doi:10.3389/fpsyg.2021.718490.

Altimir, C., & Valdés-Sánchez, N. (2020). Facial-affective communication and verbal relational offers during ruptures and resolution strategies: A systematic single case study. *Revista CES Psicología, 13*(3), 180–200. doi:10.21615/cesp.13.3.11.

Aron, L. (1996). *A Meeting of Minds. Mutuality in Psychoanalysis.* New York: Routledge.

Barros, P., Altimir, C., & Pérez, J. C. (2016). Patients' facial-affective regulation during episodes of rupture of the therapeutic alliance / Regulación afectivo-facial de pacientes durante episodios de ruptura de la alianza terapéutica. *Estudios de Psicología, 37*(2–3), 580–603. doi:10.1080/02109395.2016.1204781.

Benecke, C., & Krause, R. (2005). Facial affective relationship offers of patients with panic disorder. *Psychotherapy Research, 15*, 178–187.

Bohleber, W. (2013). The concept of intersubjectivity in psychoanalysis: Taking critical stock. *The International Journal of Psychoanalysis, 94*, 799–823.

Crits-Christoph, P., & Connolly Gibbons, M. B. (2021). Psychotherapy process–outcome research: Advances in understanding causal connections. In M. Barkham, W. Lutz, & L. G. Castonguay (Eds.), *Bergin and Garfield's Handbook of Psychotherapy and Behavior Change* (pp. 263–295). New Jersey: John Wiley & Sons, Inc.

De Maat, S., de Jonghe, F., de Kraker, R., Leichsenring, F., Abbass, A., Luyten, P., Barber, J., Van, R., & Dekker, J. (2013). The current state of the empirical evidence for psychoanalysis: A meta-analytic approach. *Harvard Review of Psychiatry, 21*, 107–137.

Ekman, P. (2007). *Emotions Revealed.* New York: St. Martin's Griffin.

Ekman, P., & Friesen, W. V. (1978). *Facial Action Coding System: A Technique for the Measurement of Facial Movement.* Palo Alto, CA: Consulting Psychologists Press.

Eubanks, C. F., Muran, J. C., & Safran, J. D. (2015). *Rupture Resolution Rating System (3RS): Manual. Technical Report.* Palo Alto, CA: Consulting Psychologists Press.

Foehl, J. C. (2010). The play's the thing. The primacy of process and the persistence of pluralism in contemporary psychoanalysis. *Contemporary Psychoanalysis, 46*, 48–86. doi:10.1080/00107530.2010.10746039.

Fonagy, P., Gergely, G., Jurist, E., & Target, M. (2002). *Affect Regulation, Mentalization and the Development of the Self.* New York: Other Press.

Fonagy, P., & Moran, G. (1993). Selecting single case research designs for clinicians. In E. N. Miller, L. Luborsky, J. P. Barber, & J. P. Docherty (Eds.), *Psychodynamic Treatment Research: A Handbook for Clinical Practice* (pp. 62–95). New York: Basic Books.

Gadamer, H. G. (1966). The universality of the hermeneutical reflection. In D. E. Linge (Ed.), *Philosophical Hermeneutics* (pp. 3–17). Berkeley: University of California Press.

Grünbaum, A. (1984). *The Foundations of Psychoanalysis: A Philosophical Critique.* Berkeley: University of California Press.

Hoffman, I. Z. (2009). Doublethinking our way to 'scientific' legitimacy: The desiccation of human experience. *Journal of the American Psychoanalytic Association, 57*(5): 1043–1069. doi:10.1177/0003065109343925.

Jiménez, J. P., & Altimir, C. (2019). Beyond the hermeneutic/scientific controversy: A case for a clinically sensitive empirical research paradigm in psychoanalysis. *The International Journal of Psychoanalysis.* doi:10.1080/00207578.2019.1636253.

Kächele, H., Schachter, J., & Thomä, H. (2012). Single-case research: The German specimen case Amalia X. In R. Levy, J. Ablon, & H. Kächele (Eds.), *Psychodynamic Psychotherapy Research. Current Clinical Psychiatry* (pp. 471–486). Totowa, NJ: Humana Press.

Kächele, H., Schachter, J., Thomä,H., & The Ulm Psychoanalytic Process Study Group. (2009). *From Psychoanalytic Narrative to Empirical Single Case Research. Implications to Psychoanalytic Practice.* New York: Routledge.

Leichsenring, F. (2005). Are psychodynamic and psychoanalytic therapies effective? A review of empirical data. *International Journal of Psycho-Analysis, 86*(3), 841–868.

Levitt, H. M. (2020). *Reporting Qualitative Research in Psychology. How to Meet APA Style Journal Article Reporting Standards.* Washington, DC: American Psychological Association.

Lyons-Ruth, K. (2000). "I sense that you sense that I sense...": Sander's recognition process and the specificity of relational moves in the psychotherapeutic setting. *Infant Mental Health Journal, 21*, 85–98. doi:10.1002/(sici)1097-0355(200001/04)21:1/2<85::aid-imhj10>3.0.co;2-f.

McLeod, J. (2011). *Qualitative Research in counseling and Psychotherapy* (2nd Ed.). London: Sage.

McWilliams, N. (2011). *Understanding Personality Structure in the Clinical Process* (2nd Ed.). New York: The Guilford Press.

Messer, S. B. (2007). Psychoanalytic case studies and the pragmatic case study method. *Pragmatic Case Studies in Psychotherapy, 3*, 55–58.

Mitchell, S. A. (1988). *Relational Concepts in Psychoanalysis. An Integration.* Cambridge: Harvard University Press.

Muran, J. C., & Eubanks, C. F. (2020). *Therapist Performance under Pressure. Negotiating Emotion, Difference, and Rupture.* Washington, DC: American Psychological Association.

Muran, J. C., Lipner, L. M., Podell, S., & Reinel, M. (2022). Rupture repair as change process and therapist challenge. *Studies in Psychology, 43*(3), 482–509. doi:10.1080/02109395.2022.2127234.

Orange, D. (2011). *The Suffering Stranger.* New York: Routledge (Taylor & Francis).

Safran, J. D. (2003). The relational turn, the therapeutic alliance, and psychotherapy research: Strange bedfellows or postmodern marriage? *Contemporary Psychoanalysis, 39*, 449–475.

Safran, J. D., & Muran, J. C. (2000). *Negotiating the Therapeutic Alliance. A Relational Treatment Guide.* New York: The Guilford Press.

Schachter, J., & Kächele, H. (2017). *Nodal Points: Critical Issues in Contemporary Psychoanalytic Therapy.* New York: IPBooks.

Schore, A. N. (2003). *Affect Regulation and the Repair of the Self.* New York: W.W. Norton & Company.

Schore, A. N. (2016). *Affect Regulation and the Origin of the Self. The Neurobiology of Emotional Development.* New York: Lawrence Erlbaum Associates, Inc.

Tuckett, D. (2004). Presidential address: Building a psychoanalysis based on confidence in what we do. *EPF Bulletin, 58*, 5–19.

Wallerstein, R. S. (1993). Psychoanalysis as science: Challenges to the data of psychoanalytic research. In N. E. Miller, L. Luborsky, J. P. Barber, & J. P. Docherty (Eds.), *Psychodynamic Treatment Research. A Handbook for Clinical Practice* (pp. 96–106). New York: Basic Books.